# *SUPERCHARGE* YOUR HEALTH!

## Other Books by Gary Null

*The Joy of Juicing*

*Nutrition and the Mind*

*Be Kind to Yourself*

*Who Are You, Really?*

*The Woman's Encyclopedia of Natural Healing*

*The Vegetarian Handbook*

# SUPERCHARGE YOUR HEALTH!

## 150 EASY WAYS TO GET STRONG, FEEL GREAT, AND LOOK YOUR BEST

....................................

## Gary Null, Ph.D.

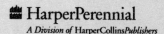
HarperPerennial
*A Division of HarperCollinsPublishers*

HarperCollins books may be purchased for educational, business, or sales promotional use. For information, please write to: Special Markets Department, HarperCollins Publishers, Inc., 10 East 53rd Street, New York, New York 10022.

*Designed by Alma Hochhauser Orenstein*

FIRST EDITION

Library of Congress Cataloging-in-Publication Data

Null, Gary.
    Supercharge your health! : 150 easy ways to get strong, feel great, and look your best / Gary Null.
    — 1st ed.
       p.  cm.
    Includes index.
    ISBN 0-06-273469-5
    1. Health behavior.  2. Health.  3. Nutrition.
  4. Exercise. I. Title.
RA776.9.N85  1997
613.7—dc21                   96-37822

97 98 99 00 01 ❖/OPM 10 9 8 7 6 5 4 3 2

# CONTENTS

# PART 1

# THINK YOUR WAY TO CHANGE

••••••••••••••••••••••

You have to go headfirst into any program for change. What I mean is, you have to first think about what you want to do, and why you want to do it. You have to think, too, about who you are, and who you want to become. Here are some ideas to get you started in this process, along with a little motivation to keep you going in your efforts to supercharge your health.

## 1 Accept responsibility for you.

*You're* responsible for your own body. It's a simple concept—one that should be obvious—but do you really feel it? Do you really understand, for instance, that unless someone's tied you to your couch, clicked on the remote, and then thrown it beyond your reach, there's no reason you have to sit there hour after hour watching TV? Do you really get the fact that unless an intruder has broken into your kitchen, put a gun to your head, and forced you to top your blueberry pie with a pint of premium ice cream, you don't have to?

The point is, the choice is always yours. What's more, you are always making choices, some healthier than others. These choices then become a pattern of behavior. Sometimes you do not like the consequences of that pattern, when, for instance, it results in overweight or disease.

But you can change your pattern. When you begin to truly accept responsibility for your health, you think of the results of your decisions and begin to make healthier choices. And as you start to look and feel better, good judgment becomes its own reward.

You'll see.

## 2 Don't take a "Band-Aid" approach to your health.

Becoming healthy is more than taking a vitamin or drinking a glass of carrot juice. You have to eliminate bad habits as you develop good ones. You can't take vitamin C and smoke a cigarette, use a B complex tablet to fight stress without trying to reduce the roots of that stress, or eat a fiber pill to counteract all the saturated fat in your diet. This simplistic "Band-Aid" approach is a game at which you will ultimately lose.

How you'll win: Develop a complete program for health and good looks that incorporates diet, exercise, and stress management, and that excludes old bad habits.

## 3  Consider why you need a program to optimize your health.

The culture of northern Italy is far different from life in America. When you go into their country, as I have, you see tiny villages alongside beautiful hills. There are eight or nine houses to a village, and villages are miles apart. Homes have been there for hundreds of years. People live well into their 80s and 90s, and remain vigorous and healthy throughout life. They do not take vitamins. Nor do they jog or take aerobics classes. Their lifestyle alone sustains good health.

Let's take a look at how these people live. If you are a northern Italian, you live a physically active life. Most of the time, you are working and moving. That, in itself, is a big plus. Second, you have a clear understanding of your life's purpose. You are happy with where you are and with what you're doing.

Third, family interaction is important. You form strong bonds in your relationships. As a result, you care about others and feel cared for in return. In addition, age is considered an asset. The older you get, the more secure you become in the knowledge that you are honored and loved by your family. Grandchildren and children look to you for guidance as they go through major life transitions. You are also the keeper of the stories and the old ways.

Further, you are self-sufficient. You do your own plumbing, your own carpentry, and your own masonry work. You have your own vineyards where you cultivate grapes, and you make wine.

You grow and harvest your own grains, and bake your own bread. You plant and harvest your own fruits and vegetables, and eat them while they are fresh. Beans and legumes are a normal part of your diet, as are seeds, nuts, olive oil, and fresh herbs.

Compare this to life in the United States. As an American, you are made, from childhood, to feel insecure about your place in the world. Family relationships are so detached that it's sometimes a wonder you don't need to wear a name tag for identification! It is rare to sit quietly without the distraction of a television, radio, or newspaper, or to enjoy the company of family members at mealtime. Work relationships are emotionally disappointing as well, as they're often competitive. As you age, your opinions and presence are no longer wanted, and you lose a sense of purpose. There is not much to expect beyond placement in a nursing home.

On the physical level, you eat so many processed foods that you don't even know what real foods taste like anymore. Stocking up on processed foods, rather than on fresh fruits and vegetables, becomes the norm. These foods are filled with excess sodium and sugar, as well as harmful colorings, preservatives, and other additives. Add to that the use of caffeine for artificial stimulation and tranquilizers to shut the brain off at night. In addition, most Americans seem to prefer sitting in front of the television set or spectator sports to any physical activity.

You can see, from these examples, two very different cultural perspectives. The Mediterranean lifestyle includes a nutrient-rich diet, an active lifestyle, and a sense of purpose throughout life. As a result, northern Italians are among the healthiest, happiest people in the world. Some Americans, unfortunately, have lost touch with their physical and psychological needs. So there is a great need for re-education on how to live.

## 4 Know the *write* way to self-understanding.

Before you embark on any program for self-improvement, it makes sense to really get to know the *self* you want to improve. A wonderful way to do this is through journal writing. By making the time to keep a journal, and jotting down thoughts, feelings, and impressions, you stimulate the process of growth and change. With every question you consider, you set into motion a dialog with your inner self. It's a purely introspective process—one that honestly reflects your feelings without the interference of outside influences. This is not to say that talking to a counselor or friend is not helpful as well. I truly believe, however, that the first step toward personal development is to get in touch with your own feelings, on your own. After all, no one knows you as well as you do.

Begin by buying a notebook for the sole purpose of keeping a personal diary. Find a quiet place where you can write for about a half hour every day. It's also a good idea to keep a memo book with you for ideas that come while you are on the move, and to keep a pad near your bed for dream messages. Keeping a pen and paper handy lets your subconscious know that you are willing to listen to messages from your innermost self.

At first, the writing process may be uncomfortable; you may even think that you can't write at all. This feeling may date back to your school days, when the focus was on parroting what the teacher said, and not on personal expression. Being criticized for sharing your unique point of view may have turned you off to penning anything more than a shopping list.

To knock out writer's block, remember that you are writing for yourself and no one else. So no one is judging you. You need to understand, too, that no one writes perfectly the first time around, not even professional writers. So just start to write and forget about not being Shakespeare. The important thing about journal-keeping is that, as you write you automatically begin to think through what you are trying to say and thoughts become clearer.

If you have a really stubborn case of writer's block, try this exercise: It's called continuous writing, and what you do is write without stopping, for three minutes. If you do not know what to say, write down, "I do not know what to say." The goal of this activity is to help you feel more comfortable with writing, and to show you that thoughts start to appear as you write. (By the way, successful professional writers use this technique, so don't waste an instant feeling silly about doing it!)

## 5 Kickstart your journal-writing with some questions.

While the exact issues you explore in your journal are uniquely yours, I have discovered over the years that most people have similar concerns. So here are some questions that frequently arise in my workshops. Answering these may help you to identify personal issues, and get you started with journal writing.

### What do you want from your work?

Make a list of the things you are looking for from a job or a career. This might include a sense of identity, enjoyment, friendships, and an opportunity to learn and grow. Does your work meet your needs? If not, what type of work might you enjoy?

### Are you happy with your home life?

Does your home give you a sense of spiritual renewal? Does it represent a retreat from the pressures of the outside world? If not, what can you do to make your home a more comfortable place? Alternatively, where would you enjoy living?

### Do you trust your intuition?

Do you pay attention to your inner voice, or do you force yourself to act the way you think you are supposed to act? Think about some hunches you have had in the past. Did you pay attention to them? If not, did you regret it? What can you do to be more in tune with your feelings?

### Do you make more commitments than you can reasonably handle?

Analyze a typical month to determine your patterns of making and keeping commitments. Notice whether you leave space for yourself.

### Are you able to say no?

Make a list of the times you said no, or wish you had. Being aware of your patterns makes it easier the next time a similar situation arises.

### What qualities do you admire in others?

Do you look up to people with courage? Compassion? Sensitivity? Open-mindedness? Do you see these qualities in yourself? If not, how can you develop them?

### Do you communicate honestly?

Do you let other people know your real needs and feelings, or do you mask them? Can you let someone know when they have hurt your feelings? If not, you are building up resentments and need to practice expressing yourself. Also, notice whether you are able to share positive thoughts and feelings with others.

These are just a few examples of the many issues you may wish to explore in your journal.

## 6 Dream on—then write it down!

Keeping a dream journal can be a useful adjunct to regular journal writing. Try it and see if it's helpful. You can easily train yourself to remember dreams by writing them down. Whatever you write—even the tiniest fragment—starts the process. You can also use a tape recorder.

Consider dreams to be messages from the unconscious that can illuminate your fears and show you where your energy is going. They can compensate for areas that are out of balance.

Many of the characters in your dreams may be facets of your own personality. Ask yourself what each one symbolizes for you, because these characters may serve in a sense as your mirror. The unfamiliar people represent the more deeply buried facets of the personality, and their behavior provides information about aspects of yourself that you have trouble visualizing.

It can be helpful to enter into a dialog with your dream characters. After you have written down the entire dream, write a letter to the characters. Ask them why they act the way they do. Why did they make that critical remark? Why are they so sad? Try to change negative outcomes or behaviors in the dream. Turn around and face your attacker. Ask someone to help you. Ask your characters what they require for health and happiness. Write all of your insights in your dream journal.

## 7 Get into goal-setting.

Once you begin getting some insight into who you are and what you want, it's time to start setting tangible goals. The importance of goals cannot be underestimated. Successful people always use them. Goals keep you focused, and your confidence increases as each small step along the way is realized.

One big plus of goal-setting—versus just drifting through life—is that it helps you come to realistic terms with time. The only thing in life you can really call your own is your time. Why waste it? Use your time wisely by paying attention to your real needs, not the superficial ones that can suck time and energy out of your life before you even know it. Determine what you want to attain, and make a plan for getting there.

## 8 Set long- and short-term goals.

First, choose a main focus. That is your long-term goal. Then create short-term goals to help you get there. And set concrete, reasonable time frames for both.

Let's use a common fitness goal—weight loss—as an example. Say you want to lose 20 pounds. That's your long-term goal. Twenty pounds seems a little intimidating, though. So what you do is give yourself a time frame of five months in which to lose the weight, and then divide the project up into short-term goals of losing a pound a week, through exercise and eating right each day. Your long-term goal thus becomes quite achievable.

## 9 Set can-do goals.

Make the goals you set attainable. Dreaming the impossible dream may sound good in a song, but dreaming the possible one will make you a whole lot happier in the end. So don't overwhelm yourself by attempting to change too much at once. Instead, make the process of change slow, but steady.

I recommend the one-bad-thing-out, one-good-thing-in approach. That is, you eliminate one bad habit at a time from your lifestyle and replace it with one good one.

For example, if you are trying to improve your

diet, you can eliminate sugar the first week, meat the second, caffeine the third, and so forth. Plus each week you can add a positive habit to your life—eating fresh fruit, for instance, or drinking enough water, or perhaps power walking or meditation. If you want to work within a more relaxed two-week time frame rather than with one-week goals, do so by all means. The point is to make your goals realistic. Tailor them to your own unique needs, desires, and personal rhythms. That way, you are sure to stick to them, and to see results.

### 10 Define success, for you.

I personally think of success not as a specific level of material accomplishment, but rather as a matter of choosing what you want out of life, and of nurturing that dream. After all, most people don't even get that far.

I also think of success as making a commitment to putting your energies to work daily. That's why I'm always telling people that they can be a success right now; they don't have to wait for some time, decades down the road, when they've finally "made it."

Today, reaffirm your choices, and then act in a way that coincides with them. When you start out with a positive thought, positive actions will naturally follow. Once you set these ideas in motion, they will become a pattern of behavior that works for you. *That's* success.

### 11 Get advice and feedback—from positive people only, please!

The process of change is an exciting one that you are probably eager to share with friends and family. Sometimes this is helpful, but not always. I say this because other people may actively discourage you from obtaining new goals. There are people who will not want to see you change. They may fear losing you as a friend, or they may realize a need for change in their own lives and not be ready to go after it. Whatever the reason, these people may try to discourage you.

I had a friend who was set on visiting Israel and Egypt. She didn't have much money, but she squirreled away whatever she could. Edith never breathed a word of her plan to anyone. After ten years of planning and saving, when she was packed and ready to go, she knocked on a neighbor's door to see if she could borrow a camera for her trip. When Edith's neighbor discovered that she was going to the Middle East, she exclaimed, "Why are you going there? Don't you know how dangerous it is?"

Edith's plan had long been set in her mind, and she wasn't one to be easily discouraged. But if you are just starting out in a new direction, a doubtful word from someone else is the last thing you need to hear.

When you do share your dreams and goals with people, look for those who offer positive support. After all, you are sharing your most cherished hopes, wishes, and dreams. It's wonderful if you have someone in your life with whom you can be honest, and yet not wind up discouraged.

You are sure to be in the company of like-minded individuals if you seek others who are pursuing similar goals. If you are serious about exercising to get into shape, joining a walking, running, or hiking club is a great idea. The people are supportive, you can get some helpful tips, and the social aspect will keep you coming back.

**12** **Realize that your friends don't necessarily want what's best for you.**

How's that again? They're your friends! Of course they want what's best for you!

Oh, they may think they do. But your friends and family may have a vested interest in the old you—the one that liked to party without noticing the fat content of the nachos, the one who appreciated all of their cooking, the one that was overweight enough not to pose a threat to them in the attractiveness area.

I'm not saying that this is always the case. You could have friends and family members that offer you nothing but genuine support. They may even be joining you and undertaking constructive life changes of their own. I'm simply saying that you should be aware of the possibility of subtle sabotage. So if someone tries to talk you out of your early-morning jog, or into an ice-cream sundae, you'll think about what may be happening. It's not that any one particular choice or incident is all that momentous, but you don't want to get into a pattern where someone close to you continually tries to undercut your health efforts out of insecurity or out of guilt about not being on a program of her or his own.

You don't have to break up your friendships over this issue. Many saboteurs don't even realize what they're doing, and you can't expect your friends to be perfect. The point is, rather, you may want to take your friends' "helpful" suggestions with a grain of salt (not literally if you're watching sodium!).

**13** **Congratulate yourself.**

As you implement your health-improvement program, acknowledge your small successes—don't look for change to happen all at once. Life is lived in small measures. If you think you haven't achieved much in life, you may not be acknowledging all the little things you have done that add up to major accomplishments.

Write down the small goals you have accomplished. How do you feel when you achieve them? With each small success, your confidence improves, allowing you to gain control of your life in other ways. One success leads to another and another.

## 14 Find out what's stopping you, and why you are allowing it.

You may have great potential but fall just short of realizing it. I have seen people with the makings of top athletes pull back and drop out the moment they start to realize their capabilities. They are afraid that once they start on the path to success their lives may never be the same. They are scared to let go of the familiar, even if it is not right for them, and to face the uncertainty on the road ahead, even if it will ultimately lead them to greater happiness.

Each day can bring something new to your life, if only you go after it. It may help to list the mental and physical roadblocks that prevent you from reaching your aim. Ask yourself, what am I afraid of giving up? What's stopping me from fulfilling my potential?

A technique for overcoming roadblocks that I find useful is visualization. When I face a conflict, I imagine a long road leading to my goal with a beautiful, beaming light at the end of it. This image reminds me that the crisis is part of a spiritual journey. As I travel this path, I notice the dragons and demons that try to stop me, but rather than focus on them, I concentrate on my heroic qualities that can provide the strength to overcome problems.

## 15 Use exercise to bust out of the low-activity/fatigue rut.

Sooner or later it happens to almost everyone—low activity and fatigue combine to form a vicious cycle that works something like this: You find yourself not feeling good for some reason, or for no particular reason, so you don't feel up to doing much. You start to mope around. Activities you once enjoyed no longer hold any interest for you, and you end up watching a lot of television. As you sit around the house, you find that you begin to eat more. And the foods you eat are unhealthy. Instead of taking the time to juice and cook, you grab some convenience food from the freezer and pop it into the microwave. Your body becomes sluggish and your thoughts defeatist.

During this period, which can last from a few days to several months, your body's caloric needs are grossly exceeded by what you take in. This means that you put more fuel into your body than it can use. Result: excess fat. And the more fat you lay down, the more sedentary you become, and the lazier you get. Now you don't have the energy to exercise. You feel trapped by increasing fatigue.

This vicious cycle keeps the body's metabolism slowed down. When your metabolism slows down, your energy diminishes. Before long, you have zero vigor; you're like a car running on two cylinders.

If you are caught in this black hole of inactivity and fatigue, don't despair. You can dig your way out. What you've got to do is start a modest, gradual exercise program that forces the body to increase its energy expenditure. As you begin to burn some of the fat and tighten some of the muscles, your mood will improve. That will motivate you to keep going forward. Instead of being caught in a vicious cycle, you'll be experiencing a *virtuous* cycle, and you'll be enjoying it! By the way, joining an exercise group or a spa may be useful. It will help you to get into a regular routine and be around positive role models.

## 16 Exercise to feel good.

Exercise increases the level of positive, feel-good hormones, known as endorphins, circulating in your brain. That helps you to sustain a good feeling throughout the day. Feeling good improves perceptions and personality, which allows you to make better and more positive choices. Studies show that, compared to the general population, runners are better able to handle psychological problems and suffer less from depression.

## 17 At the end of each day, ask yourself, "What positive choices have I made today?"

You may not have had a perfect day, and you may even have had some serious backsliding in regard to the new health habits you're trying to establish. But this happens to everybody. I'll bet that as you look back on each day's activities, you'll be able to find at least one choice you made that represented something new for you and that was life- and health-affirming. Did you choose to drink fruit juice today on your break, rather than coffee? Did you tackle those few flights of stairs, rather than take the elevator? Did you decide not to get upset about something you couldn't help today at work? Did you forego your usual banquet-style dinner and eat a salad instead? Whatever you did, feel good about it. This will help you add one more constructive change tomorrow.

**18** **Enjoy the maintenance phase of your program—it's fun!**

Here's a prediction: As you implement your body improvement plan, you will see a pattern of major effort for a couple of months—and major benefits—followed by a leveling off, a plateau of effort and benefit. When you are training for a marathon, for example, an almost yearlong project, all the major effort is in the first three, four, or five months. At first it's hard and you think, "It doesn't feel good when I wake up in the morning." "It aches when I walk." "Is it worth the pain?" Then you start looking in the mirror and seeing a body that you like. You think, "Gee, where in the world did this come from? This is something I haven't seen in a long time!" Then, it's just a matter of maintenance.

Maintenance is relatively simple. When you reach this phase, you know the routine. You know what to eat, when to eat, and how much to eat. You can start to add variety. Start cooking Mexican, Chinese, Japanese, Polynesian, Thai, Tex Mex, Cajun, French, Italian, Greek, and Caribbean: All these cuisines can be healthfully incorporated into your program.

In the area of exercise, let's say you've achieved a success plateau with power walking. Begin to extend beyond power walking to include biking, mountain climbing, cross-country skiing, or swimming. Why? Because you now know that you have the energy and strength to do these things. And because cross-training is the real athlete's key to fitness. Plus these activities are fun!

Maintenance is the fun part of your program. If you add new elements, maintenance is not boring, but rather challenging in a completely nonintimidating way. After all, once you realize, for instance, "Gee whiz, I can do a marathon—I'm in that kind of shape," then it means you can do everything less than a marathon, and easily, too. Before, the thought of going for a 10-mile run might have created a minor anxiety crisis. Now, you think it's nothing. Everything's relative.

## 19 Remember that your highs, lows, and plateaus will be unique to you.

Naturally not everybody is going to fall into a definite pattern of several months of fitness progress followed by a leveling off. Some people never seem to level off! And some make a little bit of progress, level off for a long period, and then pick up again years later. If you were to graph people's health and fitness progress, every individual's line would be different, and some would be quite complex, with alternating upturns and downturns in a whole variety of permutations. What's really important, though, is not the particular pattern a person follows, but how people on fitness programs feel compared to the time before they undertook those programs.

## 20 Know that health and vitality are within your reach at any age.

You may have heard that "you're as young as you feel." Well, I'd amend that to say "you're as young as you *do*." I believe that at 20, 30, 40, 50, 60, 70, or 80, you should be able to go white-water rafting down the Colorado River, bike riding up the coast of Maine, mountain climbing in the Rockies, or marathon running in New York City. Being physically fit at any age is possible. I know this because I have worked with older people and have helped them to reverse the diseases and conditions usually associated with aging. This has enabled many individuals to engage in competitive sports and to become world champions. I have worked with 67-year-old Thelma Wilson, 73-year-old Queenie Thompson, 55-year-old Sam Skinner, and 70-year-old Joan Rollin, all of whom went on to become world champion athletes—American national title holders.

These people need not be exceptions to the rule. By deciding how fit you want to be, maintaining a sense of focus, and taking actions necessary to achieve your goal, you can be active and healthy regardless of age.

### 21 Pick a step—any step. Then begin.

Decide today, perhaps after reading more of this book, to change something in your life, and then take a first step toward making that change. What first step do you feel comfortable taking? Don't worry if it is not the best or most appropriate step. Just begin.

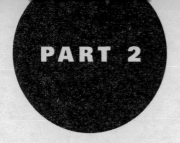

# PART 2

# EATING MADE EASY

Open up your refrigerator. Look inside your pantry. Are the items you see going to help you supercharge your health? Or are they part of the problem? The entries in this section are designed to put you on the road to healthful, enjoyable eating. First, it shows you what foods to avoid or minimize, and why. Then, it takes a look at edibles that promote well-being, focusing on the remarkable cleansing and restorative properties of fruit, vegetables, and herbs. In addition, you'll learn the easy way to keep allergies out of your life, how to eat for high energy throughout the day, and some strategies for nutritionally sound, no-hassle cooking. I welcome you to the world of health!

## 22 Beware of the typical American diet.

Before we discuss how to improve our eating habits, let's consider why we should. To do that, we have to step back and really look at the typical diet eaten in America today.

We may accept our pattern of food consumption as normal, as healthful, or even as the only way to eat, because it's ours. But take the historical perspective. It was not so long ago that food markets were lined with locally grown, fresh produce, meat from free-roaming animals, and natural foods that people would preserve at home. And while you may live under the illusion that today's mass-marketed food is equal in quality to the food of several decades ago, in reality this is far from true. Since big business got into farming, foods have carried the new burdens of pesticides, growth hormones, and preservatives. Much of our food has become processed (e.g., brown rice made branless and converted into white rice; wheat stripped of bran and germ and turned into white flour; potatoes turned into instant potato flakes, chips, and fries; and everything turned into TV dinners). This means nutrition takes a backseat to packaging and shelf-life. Also, because profit motives now cause the majority of farm animals to be fed, injected, and doused with chemicals, the meat and dairy products we consume today are full of these substances.

Junk food advertising has sold Americans on eating for entertainment, and on fast foods as a way of life. These types of foods provide a lot of sugar, saturated fat, and empty calories, but lack the vitamins and minerals necessary for optimum health.

The unfortunate bottom line: If you eat the typical American diet, you are a prime candidate for a long list of ills, ranging from allergies to cancer to heart disease. Further, the average menu is more than disruptive to your physical health: It robs you of the satisfaction that comes from preparing and eating real food.

## 23 Don't shortchange yourself nutritionally with processed foods.

Although convenience foods were originally intended as once-in-a-while replacements for cooked meals, they have become the mainstay of American life. The modern-day quicker-is-better mentality has led to a rush for convenience meals from either the supermarket or fast-food chains. Television advertising has accelerated this trend to the point where we're now a convenience-food culture.

Convenience foods are largely made up of simple (also called refined) carbohydrates. These are different from complex carbohydrates, starches, and fibers found in natural plant foods—grains, legumes, tubers, nuts and seeds, fruits, and vegetables. Simple carbohydrates are what's found in cookies, cakes, white bread, and candies—foods that have undergone processing that creates a final product unlike anything found in nature. Processing techniques, such as agitation, pressure, and extreme temperatures, strip foods of valuable vitamins and minerals.

While some companies try to return lost nutrients, they can never restore a food to its complex natural state. The label "enriched" or "fortified" is misleading because once a food's nutritional composition is destroyed, full benefit from that food can never be obtained.

And even if you benefit somewhat from the vitamins added, what about the nutrients that are not replaced? Little-understood trace elements help the body in powerful ways. Selenium, for example, helps to prevent cancer, while magnesium keeps the heart beating normally. These and other trace nutrients are not added back into refined foods.

But many chemicals *are* added. They're used to enhance the appearance, flavor, and durability of these lifeless foods. Food colorings and artificial preservatives make them look better and last longer, and lots of sugar make them palatable. Sugar also makes foods addictive, so that you keep coming back for more.

Although refined foods may seem enjoyable in the short term, eating this way over time sets you up for some serious problems. The saturated fat and excessive sugar in refined foods are linked to stomach and intestinal disorders, diabetes, hypertension, heart disease, respiratory ailments, obesity, and colon cancer. Plus chemical preservatives accelerate the aging and disease process.

In short, while convenience foods may make it a little easier on the cook, they make it a lot harder on your body.

## 24  Avoid refined sugar.

If sugar tastes so good, and supplies quick energy, then why is it bad for you?

To answer this question, we need to differentiate between sugar in its raw state and sugar after refinement. Sugar cane is full of valuable nutrients, including vitamins, minerals, essential enzymes, amino acids, fiber, and unsaturated fat. But the sugar that you eat has been stripped of everything but energy. When your cells are given energy without being fed, this disrupts metabolism, the chemical processes that take place in the body after digestion.

In an attempt to metabolize sugar, cells rob one another of vital nutrients, such as potassium, magnesium, and sodium. They also leach calcium from the skeleton, causing tooth decay and dry, brittle bones. As a result of all this, body systems can break down and become receptive to a number of diseases. Sugar consumption has been linked to diabetes, hypoglycemia, dental caries, osteoporosis, behavioral disorders, obesity, heart disease, strokes, stomach problems, and premature aging.

The energy boost that manufacturers advertise is only temporary. Sugar consumption raises blood sugar for just a few minutes, and is quickly followed by a rapid drop. For some people this can mean hypoglycemia, or low blood sugar, characterized by headaches, dizziness, fatigue, or irritability. Studies show that sugar is actually a poor source of energy that lowers performance within an hour of being consumed.

Our natural love for sugar is nature's enticement to reach for succulent, nourishing fruits packed with vitamins, nutrients, and fiber. Just a small amount of fruit is enough to satisfy a sweet craving. But the isolated substance offered by industry does not satisfy in the same way. Just think about it. How many bananas can you eat? How many candy bars? Sugar, once refined, becomes addictive. Food manufacturers know this and add it to practically every food they market. While you would expect to find sugar in cookies, other desserts, and soft drinks, it is also a hidden ingredient in soups, frozen vegetables, spaghetti sauce, ketchup, and salad dressings. Small wonder that the average American consumes 150 pounds of sugar per year. Nor is it surprising that America has become a chronically sick nation.

### 25 Beware of "sweet deceits."

To deceive consumers into thinking they are getting less sugar, companies manufacturing processed foods disguise the sweetener by referring to various forms of it on their product labels, such as corn syrup, glucose, sucrose, fructose, maple syrup, or honey. When several of these names appear on a food label, it looks as if there are a variety of different ingredients, but they're all basically forms of sugar, and sugar may well be the product's main ingredient. The next time you're in the supermarket, pick up a jar or box of food and read the label. You may be surprised to see just how much sugar manufacturers actually use.

### 26 Become sweetener savvy.

As you cut down on or eliminate sugar, you should know that even relatively healthful honey and maple syrup can be chemically treated, over-processed, and overused, contributing to the same sugar-induced diseases that white sugar does. If you do buy these foods, make sure they are pure, and use them sparingly.

Artificial sweeteners are no solution. Saccharin is linked to cancer, aspartame to seizures, and sorbitol to fructose intolerance, as well as kidney and liver problems. By the way, artificial sweeteners haven't really made a dent in sugar consumption. Over the years, surveys have shown steady rises in both sugar and sugar substitute sales. The only solution is to stay away from refined sugar and sugar substitutes completely, and to retrain your taste buds to enjoy nature's rich storehouse of unrefined foods.

### 27 Forget the maxim that meat and dairy are essential to good health.

When you grew up, meat and dairy products were probably being touted as the be-all and end-all of good nutrition. But we know more now. So if meat and dairy are still mainstays of your diet, you may consider eating less of these foods once you realize that too much animal protein is unhealthy, and once you learn that you do not need to rely on these foods as your sole source of protein.

Let's begin by looking at the hazards to your health. Countless studies confirm that diets high in animal products contribute to heart disease and many types of cancer, including cancer of the breast, colon, prostate, pancreas, kidney, and endometrium. This knowledge has prompted the American Heart Association to recommend that Americans cut down on meat. The government is also suggesting that the standard diet include less dairy, as well as less fat and oil, and more grains, fruits, and vegetables.

Food poisoning from meat and dairy is another serious health hazard that has been on the rise in recent years. It stems from highly toxic bacteria, such as *E. coli* and salmonella, which find their way into beef, poultry, pork, eggs, milk, and cheese. Each year, millions become sickened by these foods, and many perish. Especially susceptible are children, the elderly, and people with weak immune systems. In 1993, this problem was given media attention when 500 people were hospitalized with *E. coli* from hamburgers eaten at a Seattle, Washington, Jack-in-the-Box restaurant. Three children died as a result. The meat industry promised to look into the matter, but the problem continues.

If you think of meat and dairy as your prime source of protein, you need to realize that other sources are equally good, if not better. For centuries, people around the world have combined grains and vegetables, and have eaten soy products, seeds, and nuts, for their primary protein sources.

## 28 Don't overdo the protein!

From advertising, and from outdated nutrition education, one could get the idea that we're all in danger of suffering from a protein deficiency. This is not true. What is true is that protein is the main building material for muscles, blood, skin, hair, nails, and organs. It is needed to form hormones, enzymes, and antibodies, and can be a source of heat and energy. It's also necessary for proper elimination.

But it doesn't follow from this that if protein is so important, more must be better. Actually, more is not better. Most people eat twice as much protein as their body requires. Since protein is not storable, your body excretes what it does not use right away. That means extra work for your kidneys. Eating too much protein has another disadvantage. It lessens your appetite for fruits and vegetables, causing you to miss out on essential nutrients and fiber.

## 29 Go back to school about protein.

You may have heard people refer to complete protein. A complete protein food is one containing all eight essential amino acids not produced by the body. (Amino acids are organic compounds that are needed to form proteins. Humans have 22 amino acids inside them, but eight of these are not manufactured by the body and must be obtained from food.) In the meat-and-potatoes days of American cuisine, it used to be taught that meat products were the only sources of complete protein. But we now know that other foods contain a full spectrum of amino acids as well. These are the soy products: soybeans, soy flour, tempeh, and tofu. Soy flour, in fact, contains more protein than meat.

It also used to be taught that in order to get

complete protein from nonmeat sources, you had to eat certain foods together at one meal, for example, grains and legumes, or grains and dairy. The latest research, though, shows that this planned protein-combining at a given meal is unnecessary. By eating a variety of high-quality nonmeat sources of protein, and eating enough of them, you can get all the protein you need. And this can be done even without dairy products, as other cultures have shown us.

### 30 Cut your fat intake—but don't eliminate it altogether.

A small amount of fat in the diet is essential to health. It keeps your body warm and provides you with energy. Plus fat-soluble vitamins A, D, E, and K need it to help them work. Fat produces hormones, keeps skin healthy, and slows down the aging process. Last but not least, it protects your heart, nerves, blood vessels, and internal organs.

The problem with the American diet is that it contains too much fat. Generally, a diet that's 10 to 15 percent fat, which translates into 1 to 2 tablespoons of fat daily, is all you need, while the average person eats a diet that's 45 percent fat. Most of this fat is saturated, which contributes to a variety of problems that plague the American population, including obesity, cardiovascular problems, circulatory disorders, gastrointestinal diseases, and free-radical damage. While there is a place in the diet for both saturated and unsaturated fats, the key is to keep the consumption of both minimal, and to focus on the unsaturated variety.

Examples of good natural sources of unsaturated fat are baked salmon, broiled tuna, and raw sunflower seeds.

### 31 Stay away from saturated fat—it's solid.

You don't have to be mystified about dietary fat. It's all very simple: Saturated fat, a prime American dietary downfall, generally stays solid at room temperature. It's found in butter, lard, the fatty part of meat, fries, and commercially made cookies, doughnuts, cakes, and pies. Unsaturated fat, the better kind, usually remains liquid at room temperature. It's found in unrefined oils such as canola, soy, safflower, and olive. Other sources include grains, legumes, nuts, and seeds.

### 32 Remember that "unsaturated fats" are not all alike.

When shopping for unsaturated fats, beware of labels that read "hydrogenated." This tells you that the product came from an unsaturated source but that it is now saturated. It also means that it is adulterated with chemical preservatives, coloring agents, and flavors that make it harmful to your health.

### 33 Avoid the drug in a mug: caffeine.

Which is why, the next time you're offered a cup of coffee, you should "just say no!" You see, although it's only a mild stimulant to the central nervous system, over time caffeine becomes an addictive drug. Many Americans abuse caffeine without even knowing it, and suffer from withdrawal when they miss a dose. You may think you are drinking a cup of coffee only because you enjoy it, but try skipping a cup. You may experience headaches, drowsiness, loss of concentration, and even constipation.

Although it is most commonly associated with

coffee, caffeine is also found in teas (with the exception of many herbal teas), chocolate, colas, and stay-awake and headache medications.

Caffeine can lead to a wide array of medical complications, although its effects vary widely from person to person. The problems it can cause or contribute to include insomnia, heart stress, gastrointestinal disorders, osteoporosis, nervous system disorders, and even cancer. Clinical experience shows that pancreatic cancer, which kills tens of thousands of Americans each year, has a statistical connection to coffee intake. Drinking more than five cups a day triples your risk, while abstaining from coffee completely lowers your chance to almost zero.

By the way, do you think caffeine addiction is a problem for adults only? You may be surprised to learn just how much caffeine many children consume. While a single cup of coffee contains 30 to 100 milligrams of caffeine, a 12-ounce can of cola has 35 to 55 mg. So children who drink a few colas a day are drinking as much caffeine as many adult coffee drinkers.

### 34 Don't overwork your adrenals with caffeine and sugar.

Are your adrenal glands overstimulated? If so, you may be exhausted a lot of the time. You see, these organs, which sit atop each kidney, are meant to supply you with the "fight or flight" hormones necessary for protection.

The trouble is, this personal protection system is often unable to differentiate between major and minor problems. The adrenals are unable to say, "hold on a second, this is really not so important that I should be secreting this adrenaline and exhausting you. Why don't you just take a couple of deep breaths and get a new perspective on the situation?" Instead, every worry, no matter how small, leads to stress and exhaustion.

The problem of adrenal overload is amplified if you artificially stimulate the adrenal glands with caffeine and sugar. And that's what most people do. They routinely start the day with a cup of coffee, artificial orange juice, and some sugar-coated cereal, none of which were designed to be used by your body. What happens is that the adrenal glands become so worn down that people depend upon these stimulants to start the day. We're all familiar with the commercial that tells us the best part of waking up is having a particular brand of coffee in our cup. And here I was thinking that the best part of waking up was being alive! Alas, most people are dependent on coffee and unable to start the day without it.

## 35 Stop accepting the "acceptable poison": alcohol.

Think about alcohol's image in our society. It's generally pictured as a normal and positive aspect of adult life, isn't it? We're supposed to use it to unwind after a hard day, to celebrate life's happy occasions, and to complement good meals. Characters on TV programs are shown incorporating alcoholic beverages into their daily lives in a glamorous and fun-filled way that can make a viewer want to follow suit.

But the easy acceptance of alcohol in our society is unfortunate, considering all we know of its detrimental effects. Alcohol is an addictive poison that can gradually become an obsession. When that happens, it ruins your life and the lives of people around you. What's more, even small amounts impair judgment, concentration, and coordination, as witnessed by the many automobile accidents that occur while the drivers are under alcohol's influence.

The devastating effects of drinking are at first difficult to see, especially if you're the one doing the drinking. Initially, you feel stimulated, even euphoric, as social inhibitions become relaxed. Eventually, the feeling wears off, and alcohol's true depressant effects are felt as the brain shuts down. Next morning's hangover causes you to suffer from headache, nausea, and exhaustion. What's happening is that your liver is working overtime to remove toxins from your system. At the same time, your kidneys act as a diuretic and eliminate more water than they take in, resulting in dehydration.

You have probably heard of the dangers of serious drinking. Alcoholism becomes a fatal addiction that kills its victims via cirrhosis of the liver, cancer, and brain damage. What you may not know is that occasional drinking can be just as deadly. Recent studies link as few as three drinks a week to cancer of the breast, oral cavity, esophagus, pharynx, and larynx.

### 36 You must remember this. . .

. . . It's good nutrition in a nutshell: Generally, a healthy diet is high in complex (not refined) carbohydrates, with smaller amounts of protein and fat (which should be primarily unsaturated as opposed to saturated).

### 37 Make complex carbohydrates three-quarters of your diet.

Complex carbohydrates are essential to good health. They are excellent sources of energy that your body can either use right away or store. They also contain cellulose, a fibrous material that helps in the elimination process. Moreover, complex carbohydrates increase metabolism, and are full of essential vitamins, minerals, and amino acids.

Note that complex carbohydrates are often confused with simple carbohydrates, found in refined foods such as white bread and cake. In truth, the complex variety burn slowly so that the dieter is satisfied with less food and the diabetic's blood sugar remains stable longer. Learn to distinguish between the two: Complex carbohydrates have nutritional merit, and empty starches and sugars have lost their value through refinement.

Sources of complex carbohydrates: grains—a group that ranges from the familiar whole wheat and brown rice to the lesser known but highly nutritious quinoa, spelt, and amaranth; legumes— e.g., lentils, black beans, peanuts, and the invaluable group of soy products, such as tofu, tempeh, and miso; vegetables—everything from artichokes to dandelion greens to potatoes to zucchini; fruits— from the tiny, such as cherries, to the tremendous, such as watermelon, they're wonders of nutrition and detoxification; and nuts and seeds (eat these in lesser quantities than the others).

## 38 Play the three magic keys to health: VEGETABLES, VEGETABLES, VEGETABLES!

Okay, maybe I've oversimplified, but vegetables are certainly vital to a healthy, long life. And there does seem to be something almost magical in the way they combine a variety of life-giving benefits. So let's go beyond three keys to health—let's name 30. If I were to name 30 "magic" vegetables to include in a diet, I would list the following:

**ALFALFA.** Alfalfa sprouts, in a salad or juiced, are rich in calcium, potassium, iron, and magnesium.

Alfalfa is one of the finest blood-cleansing foods you can use. In folk medicine, taking the juice of alfalfa is linked to helping with arthritis, gout, and indigestion.

**ARUGULA.** A common green used in Italy that is gaining popularity in this country. It's rich in calcium, vitamin A, and iron.

**AVOCADO.** A good source of the healthy fats that you need in your diet.

**BEET GREENS.** Great for juicing, and loaded with healing enzymes.

**BEETS.** These build blood because they are rich in iron. Also, they're rich in magnesium and vitamin A. Beet leaves and beet root constitute one of the most popular forms of juice, especially when combined with celery and cucumber.

**BROCCOLI.** Proven anticancer and cleansing properties.

**BRUSSELS SPROUTS.** Also has anticancer and detoxification effects.

**CABBAGE.** Raw cabbage juice, three times a day, has been used to heal ulcers, calm the gastrointestinal system, and stimulate proper digestion. Has antiviral and antibacterial qualities.

**CARROTS.** The always healthful carrot is one of the best foods for your eyes and your immune system because of its beta carotene.

**CAULIFLOWER.** A cruciferous vegetable valuable to your immune health. The cruciferous group of vegetables, which also includes cabbage, broccoli, and Brussels sprouts, are terrific for you because they contain cancer-blocking compounds called indoles. To make them taste great, remember not to overcook—try steaming them lightly.

**CELERY.** One of nature's perfect diuretics, which means that it helps rid your system of excess water. Four ounces of celery juice combined with 4 ounces of cucumber juice and apple juice is a great liver flush, kidney flush, and energizer. It also helps with digestion, and is known to lower blood pressure.

**CHICORY.** A blood purifier that stimulates the liver and kidneys to detoxification.

**COLLARD GREENS.** Common item in the South, but not anywhere else in the country. They should be, though, because they provide a whole gamut of minerals, and are an outstanding nondairy source of calcium. Collard greens have been used to treat arthritis and urinary infections, and for blood cleansing.

**DANDELION GREENS.** One of the most nutrient-rich, low-calorie foods anywhere. Historically, the juice of the dandelion has been used as a liver detoxifier; it is also a very good source of calcium, magnesium, and potassium.

**EGGPLANT.** Rich in cholesterol-lowering nutrients. Also a good source of essential fatty acids. Helps with digestion.

**GARLIC.** Lowers your blood pressure and cholesterol (if that's what your body needs). Has natural antibacterial, antiviral, and antiyeast properties.

**KALE.** It's rich in minerals and vitamins and has anticancer properties. Kale probably has more calcium than any of the other greens, with the exception of sea vegetables. It's also high in magnesium. Put into a juice or stir-fried with olive oil, garlic, onion, and cayenne pepper, it's a delicious dish.

**MUSHROOMS.** Reishi, shiitake, and maitake mushrooms stimulate the immune system. The Chinese and others in the Orient have used them for thousands of years as medicines; these mushrooms have powerful antitumor, antibacterial, and antiviral properties. In addition, they help to lower cholesterol.

**MUSTARD GREENS.** Used for centuries throughout the South, they are a primary source of calcium,

beta carotene, and other minerals. Good for detoxification.

**ONIONS.** An onion a day helps keep a heart
attack away. They can lower blood pressure and
cholesterol. Onions are also antibacterial and antiviral. They counter asthma, colds, and the flu.

**PARSLEY.** This green should be more than just a
decoration. Juicing parsley makes it one of the great
adrenal-gland stimulators for energy. It is also
excellent for treating any form of infection, and it
has anticancer properties.

**PEAS.** Peas are powerful intestinal cleansers, and
they can lower "bad" cholesterol.

**PEPPERS.** Red, green, and yellow peppers are
great sources of vitamin C, frequently containing as
much as an orange, without the acidity. They are
high in minerals, and have anticancer properties.

**POTATOES.** You may not appreciate the importance of potatoes, and think of them only as a
starch. Yes, there's starch there, but it's a healthy
starch. Potatoes are good if you need your blood
sugar balanced, or are suffering from diabetes or
hypoglycemia. They also have natural antiviral
properties.

**RADISHES.** The radish family are natural diuretics. Good for liver flushes.

**SPINACH.** In small amounts, spinach is healthy
because of its iron content. The reason you should
not be eating Popeye-sized portions is that spinach
is high in oxalic acid, which can chelate out calcium and zinc from your system.

**STRING BEANS.** Good for cleansing the liver.

**SWISS CHARD.** Swiss chard is not eaten by many
people, and that's too bad. It's a delicious green,
and it's rich in calcium and potassium. If you have
problems with constipation, it acts as a natural laxa-
tive.

**TOMATOES.** Tomatoes are known to have anticancer properties. These delights of the garden are rich in beta carotene.

**WATERCRESS**. Extraordinarily rich source of chlorophyll, sulfur, and iodine. Has primarily been used as a blood detoxifier for people who have underactive thyroids.

### 39 Think plant.

When in doubt about what to eat, think plant. Plant-food-centered meals, properly prepared, provide a full spectrum of your basic requirements: proteins, essential fatty acids, complex carbohydrates, vitamins, and minerals. Plus it's the plant food in your meals—never the animal—that provides you with ever-important fiber. Going beyond meals, fresh vegetable juices and supplements can provide you with extra power.

One of the reasons you should think plant when you eat is that our bodies seem to have been designed for the herbivorous—as opposed to the carnivorous—way of life. Consider human teeth. Unlike the sharp, fanglike teeth of truly carnivorous animals, used to tear meat from bone, most of our teeth are the flat, grinding kind useful in processing plant foods. Our digestive tracts as well are more suited to plants; they're long. The true carnivore's digestive tract is much shorter than ours, enabling the meat-eating animal to process its food in a short time, before it putrefies and causes damage.

Plus we meat- and dairy-loving Americans can no longer ignore the mountain of studies that have come out linking consumption of these foods—and the hormones and antibiotics they're laced with—to various forms of cancer, as well as to heart disease. Or we can ignore this research at our own peril, because the studies, published in respected scientific peer-reviewed journals, have been piling up for years now and all lead to the same conclusion—for human well-being, plant food is best.

Many people these days go beyond that in their thinking; concerned with animal well-being, they ask, why kill other creatures for food if we don't have to? There's also the question of our planet's welfare, and all its peoples'. When plant food is eaten directly by people, you have a vastly more efficient protein-delivery system than when it is fed first to cattle, which are then used for food. Did you know that to produce one pound of meat, it takes 16 pounds of grain? If we're concerned about feeding people economically, saving Earth's precious forest lands, and saving water too, a plant-based diet makes the most sense.

## 40 Drink fresh vegetable juice for concentrated nourishment.

If you want to treat your body to a variety of life-enhancing nutrients, there's no better way to go than with freshly made juice. Sure, you could get some of the vitamins and minerals found in vegetables from a multivitamin pill. But here's what you wouldn't be getting: the numerous disease-blocking phytochemicals—substances researchers are only beginning to understand—found in each and every vegetable. You'd also be missing out on valuable enzymes, amino acids, and trace elements. Plus juice is more digestible, and tastier, than a pill. In short, by drinking juice you're flooding your body with the best that nature has to offer in the way of healing power, and doing it deliciously.

I recommend starting out in the morning with a large glass (12 ounces) of juice. You might want to make your day's supply at this time and keep the rest in the refrigerator, in a sealed container. A Champion juicer does a nice job.

What to include in your juice? Use mostly vegetables, although watermelon is wonderful. Other fruits that are good in moderation are berries, pears, and grapefruit. Good base vegetables for your mixed juice are celery, cucumber, and cabbage, because they contain a lot of water. Vegetables that contain little water, such as parsley, spinach, and dandelion greens, are stronger on the system and should be diluted with water (use 10 parts water to 1 part of these strong juices). A caveat on carrots—they contain a lot of sugar, so be careful with them if you have diabetes or hypoglycemia.

Don't overlook sprouts, such as alfalfa, in your juice mixtures; they're nutritional bonanzas. Do use organic vegetables and fruits whenever possible. You don't want to be drinking pesticides; they're hormone mimickers that can create imbalances in your system, which may eventually result in disease. And since the whole idea of juicing is maximizing health and avoiding disease, organic produce should be your choice.

## 41 Don't miss miso.

This nutritionally superior food has been helping people to better health for thousands of years. Miso is a fermented product made from soybeans. Like yogurt, its bacteria do good work in your intestines—a real plus because the health of your intestines determines the health of your body. But do use miso sparingly because of its high sodium content.

## 42 Eat seaweed.

Eat seaweed? Am I kidding? Not at all. Sea vegetables are loaded with minerals. They should be included in the diet because they offer micronutrients that land-grown foods no longer contain, due to soil depletion. Sea vegetables have names that include kombu, wakami, nori, and hijiki. They are bought dry and can be stored for months. Flaked, cooked sea vegetables are a great addition to casseroles or soups. Add some to miso soup for a new kind of nutritional boost.

## 43 Use sprouts for a great nutrition source—and a fun project.

Everyone interested in maximizing health should be familiar with sprouts. These are simply a power-house of nutrition; you just cannot find anything healthier, and they work to cleanse as well as nour-ish. Health food stores and supermarkets are stocked with a variety of these super foods, although you might want to buy them in seed form and grow your own at home. It's a little more work that way, but growing your own sprouts is an enjoyable project that will save you money and guarantee freshness.

It's really easy! Just place 2 tablespoons of alfalfa seeds, or ¼ cup of mung beans or lentils, in a quart jar. Add water, and soak seeds for a few hours or overnight, covered. Then drain; you can use a cheesecloth secured to the jar rim with a rubber band to keep the seeds from escaping. Rinse seeds.

For the next four days, rinse the seeds twice daily. Each time you return them to the jar, seal it with a cheesecloth or other screen and invert the jar over a dish rack, so that the water can drain out.

On day four, rinse your sprouts. Soak them in water and skim off the hulls that float to the sur-face. Put sprouts in a container in direct or indirect sunlight, and soon they'll develop chlorophyll. They'll turn green!

Enjoy your sprouts in salads, soups, sandwiches,

or casseroles. (You can refrigerate them, dry, for 1 to 2 weeks.)

## 44 Learn about herbs.

Herbs are good medicine—and more. They have been used medicinally since long before recorded history began. Originally, generations of trial and error taught prehistoric people which plants to use when treating injuries and diseases. Life-saving knowledge was passed down through the ages and survives to some degree in every culture today.

In relatively recent times, Western civilization has sought to substitute chemicals for natural medicines. The tide began to turn in the 1600s when the Church of Rome voiced its objection to pagan wisdom, and the Swiss physician Paracelsus began to use inorganic cures like mercury and antimony. Soon chemical-based medicine became a monopoly, one that's lasted to the present. While some chemical-based medicines are effective and even life-saving in their curative abilities, their misuse and overuse has resulted in problematic side effects, both for individuals and on a societal level. For example, the overuse of antibiotics causes candidiasis in individuals, as well as the emergence of new drug-resistant "super-bugs" that threaten whole populations.

As the limitations of modern medicines become increasingly apparent, people are once again turning their interest to natural remedies. Individuals who experience herbal healing have confidence in the effectiveness of herbs to cure without dangerous side effects. Scientists around the world, in a desperate search for answers to AIDS, cancer, and other conditions not cured by standard medicine, have begun to study the properties of herbs, and are amazed at their immune-enhancing effects. Astragalus and licorice have powerful anticancer properties, for example, while echinacea and gold-enseal taken at the first sign of a cold or flu will help lessen its severity.

Of course herbs are more than medicine. They are foods that nourish, spices that enliven, and teas that soothe and delight. In the ninth century, Charlemagne grew herbs in his royal kitchen and called them the friends of physicians and the praise of cooks. Why not experiment with aromatic herbs and spices for their subtle and delicious tastes? End the meal with an herbal tea that helps digestion, like spearmint or peppermint, instead of a caf-feinated brew that drains the system. If it's energy you're after, try ginseng. It promotes alertness and vigor without the coffee jitters.

**45** **Learn how to use herbs.**

Here are some herbs you can try for their bene-ficial effects, or just for taste. Familiarize yourself with natural flavorings. Work with various season-ings and, in a short time, you will know just how much to use to create a delectable meal.

**HERBS AND SPICES: THEIR USES AND BENEFITS\***

| Herb or Spice | Can Enhance | Health Benefits |
| --- | --- | --- |
| Allspice | Soups, vegetables, baked goods | Relieves indigestion |
| Basil | Salads, eggs, dressings | Helps gastric problems |
| Cayenne | Curries, chili powders, eggs, sauces | Great for heart; stops bleeding |
| Cloves | Stewed fruit, chutneys | Oil stops toothache |
| Dill | Potatoes, green beans | Calms upset stomach |

| Herb or Spice | Can Enhance | Health Benefits |
| --- | --- | --- |
| Fennel | Salads, rice, potatoes, lentils | Arouses appetite; relieves stomach cramps |
| Garlic | Vegetables, dressings, meats | Builds immunity against infections and colds; great for the heart |
| Ginger | Dressings, Oriental dishes, stews, baked goods | Promotes cleansing through perspiration |
| Horseradish | Cream sauces, cooked vegetables, cheese dips, salad dressings | Stimulates circulation, good for rheumatic problems |
| Marjoram | Tomato dishes and sauces, green beans, minestrone soup | Herbal pillow may help rheumatism |
| Parsley | Soups, stews, gravies | Diuretic |
| Rosemary | Stuffing, rice, salad dressings, sauces | Promotes digestion; too much may be unsafe |
| Sage | Grains, soups, chowders | Reduces perspiration |
| Thyme | Bread dough, stuffing, gumbos, brown sauce | Tincture helps bronchial problems |

*This is not meant to take the place of a doctor's advice.

**46** **Consider herbs for your nerves.**

These 10 herbs, which can be enjoyed in tea form, have traditionally been used in restoring brain and nervous system stability. (A health-care practitioner trained in herbal medicine can steer you toward the herbs most suited to your particular needs.)

**PASSION FLOWER.** Tones the sympathetic nervous system and is good for insomnia, restlessness, and nervous headaches. Steep 5 to 15 minutes. Drink one cup per day.

**VALERIAN ROOT.** Strong sedative and nerve tonic that helps alleviate painful emotional stress. Note: Large dosages can bring on depression. Simmer 3 ounces for 3 to 15 minutes and drink three times daily.

**WOOD BETONY.** Excellent for calming the nerves and cleansing the liver. This remedy helps alleviate headaches and nervous twitching of the face. Historically used to treat insanity, neuralgia, colds, and cramps. Steep 3 ounces 5 to 15 minutes and drink once or twice a day.

**CHAMOMILE.** Counters insomnia and nervousness, especially when due to a weak stomach. When combined with cramp bark, chamomile is a traditional remedy for hysteria. Steep flowers 10 to 30 minutes and drink once a day.

**GOTU KOLA.** Valued for the treatment of depression, blood diseases, and mental weakness. Gotu kola neutralizes blood acids and is known as a longevity herb. When combined with a small amount of goldenseal, its brain tonic properties are further enhanced. Steep for 5 to 15 minutes and drink once a day.

**SKULLCAP.** Soothes the nervous system in several ways. It can assist in breaking an addiction to drugs, such as barbiturates and Valium. When ½ ounce of skullcap is combined with ¼ ounce of American ginseng, it is a good treatment for alcoholism. Mixed with lady's slipper, it acts as a tonic for hysteria and headaches. For the best effects, skullcap should be as fresh as possible when used.

Skullcap can be made into a tea by steeping for 15 to 30 minutes and can be taken once daily.

**HAWTHORN BERRIES.** Known primarily as a heart tonic, hawthorn tea is also good for nervous conditions and insomnia. Simmer berries 5 to 15 minutes and drink 1 cup two to three times daily.

**MOTHERWORT.** Helps all nervous conditions, cramps, convulsions, and sleeplessness. Steep 5 to 15 minutes and drink three to four times a day.

**HOPS.** Promotes sleep when insomnia is a problem. Steep 5 to 15 minutes and drink once a day.

**BLESSED THISTLE.** Improves digestion and circulation. As a brain food, blessed thistle helps to stimulate memory and relieve headaches. Pour boiling water over the herb and allow to steep for 5 to 15 minutes. Drink as needed.

WARNING: Do not take blessed thistle alone or in large quantities during pregnancy.

### 47 Tailor your dietary changes for you.

Some people can plunge right in to a completely new pool of dietary ways, feel fine about it, and never look back. But most people can't. If they try to make too many changes at once, they get discouraged and revert to their old habits. If you are like most people, don't feel bad: just make your changes in steps.

As I mentioned before, I recommend a two-at-a-time, one-bad-choice-out, one-good-choice-in approach to improved health. By doubling up like this you're making real progress, but you're not overwhelmed by the process.

Think of a yearlong health-improvement process. If I said, right off the bat, "Look, your eating habits are awful; you need to make at least 50 changes," you would be discouraged from the outset. But with one positive item added every two weeks, and one negative one subtracted, you will be accomplishing a lot, in easily doable steps.

Just remember, once the bad is out, it should not come back, and once the good is in, it's in to stay. So if you decide to make fresh juice, then juicing should become a part of your daily routine. If you begin to eat salads, then you should eat them daily. If you stick with your new patterns, by the end of the year you'll have completed 52 substantial changes—26 bad items out and 26 good items in. As a result, you'll be totally revitalized.

### 48 Detoxify.

Detoxification is the first step to a healthier body, and it all starts with dietary modification. Here's how to eat to cleanse your system. Again, make these changes in steps if that's easier for you.

First, avoid alcohol, caffeine, and refined sugars. Second, up your water intake. Third, keep in mind that whenever you eat meat or dairy, you are taking in any number of drugs that have been given to the animals these foods are from. In addition, these foods contain high levels of saturated fat, which traps poisons that get into the system. So you're going to want to eliminate or, at the very least, cut down on animal products when you're in the detox process.

In place of these products, eat a fruit- and vegetable-based diet, and drink fresh juices. As you prepare your meals, remember that organic food is best. This is food grown or raised without synthetic fertilizers, pesticides, or drugs. In other words, it's the cleanest food you can get, which is certainly what you want as you cleanse your system. (Note: Some products are labeled *natural*, but that doesn't necessarily mean they were grown organically.)

Foods promoting better digestion include pears, blueberries, strawberries, and papaya; apples are a wonderful colon cleanser and an overall tonic as well. Of course, don't limit yourself to these; the important thing is to think plant—as opposed to processed—foods. This may be a big menu shift for you, but once you start eating these health-givers from the earth, your tastes will change for the better in no time at all.

### 49 Your body is over two-thirds water—drink like it!

Drinking lots of cool, clear water isn't just necessary for detoxification. It's necessary for life. And the emphasis should be on *clear*—your drinking water should be as pure as possible, free of fluoride, chlorine, metals, bacteria, and viral contaminants. All these substances may be affecting you negatively without your even suspecting it. You can buy a simple, inexpensive purification system for your home that will draw out harmful additives.

By the way, thirst isn't always a reliable guide to how much you should drink. Include eight glasses of water, 8 to 10 ounces each, every day, and drink them between, rather than with, meals.

### 50 Change your eating patterns for optimal energy.

Are most of your days marked by an energy deficit? Sometimes, getting more energy into your life may be as simple as modifying your food consumption pattern. If you're one of the millions of Americans who skips breakfast, has a small lunch, and eats the major meal of the day at dinner, you're fueling your body in the least intelligent way imaginable. No offense meant—the point is that changing your meal pattern, as well as being conscientious about food choices within each meal, can really make a difference in how you feel during all your waking hours.

Start the day with some juice, preferably vegetable juice to get the enzyme action going, to get cleansing chlorophyll, to get the antioxidants that fight for you, and to get the vitamins and minerals that build your body in countless ways. These act as the spark plugs for your body so that you're functioning on all cylinders.

Follow that with a good, healthy breakfast. If you skip this meal you are setting yourself up for failure, as research indicates people who miss breakfast tend to be overweight. Give yourself quality protein—either a hot grain cereal, eggs, or a protein drink made from rice or soy protein powder. Any of these will give your body the raw materials it needs to keep your muscles working from breakfast to lunch.

Lunch should be your major meal of the day. Soup is a good choice, or, if you wish, fish, salad, vegetables, grains, or legumes. Select foods that you enjoy, but beware of high-calorie dressings and sauces.

For dinner, have a light meal so that you feel refreshed and energetic enough to enjoy the evening. If you eat too much you will just sit in front of the television like a zombie. Your dinner can be something as simple as a large salad with a baked potato, a lean piece of fish with a salad, or pasta with salad and whole grain bread. Just remember, the lightest meal of the day is supper.

Avoid snacking after dinner, as you don't want to fill up the ol' belly just before bedtime. If you should get hungry, try carbonated water with a twist of lemon or lime, or a small fruit.

## 51 Energize your day right from the beginning—with a proper breakfast.

Normal energy in an adult or teenager starts in the morning with a proper breakfast, e.g., a whole-grain cereal, fresh fruit, and a milk substitute such as rice milk, soy milk, or even almond milk (all of which look, smell, and taste like cow's milk, but do not have any of that substance's allergenic potential). With this breakfast, the body has what it needs to get it through the morning on an even keel, and to repair and rebuild the system.

I like to invent energizing hot breakfast combos, and you might want to follow suit. Here are a couple of mine to get you started.


### ALMOND CINNAMON MILLET

*6 ounces millet*

*1 ½ ounces almonds, blanched and chopped*

*Pinch of cinnamon*

Cook millet in a saucepan in 13 ounces water. When water comes to a boil, lower heat and cook until water is absorbed. Stir occasionally. Add remaining ingredients. Mix well.

SERVES 1.


### OLD-FASHIONED WHEAT BREAKFAST

*6 ounces cream of wheat*

*1 tablespoon maple syrup*

*1 ½ ounces brewer's yeast*

*1 banana, mashed*

Cook cream of wheat in 12 ounces of water for 10 minutes. Stir occasionally over medium heat. Add remaining ingredients.

SERVES 1.

**SUPERCHARGE YOUR HEALTH!**

### 52 Avoid the blood sugar blues.

Are you in the sugary-snack habit? Get out of it. Putting more glucose, or sugar, into the bloodstream than the body can handle on a regular basis can cause unhealthy fluctuations in blood sugar.

This is how it happens. You raise the blood sugar to very high levels with a sugary food or drink. One large glass of orange juice, for instance, has more available glucose than you generally have circulating in your blood. The body then asks the pancreas to issue insulin—a hormone that acts to regulate sugar metabolism—to lower the sugar influx.

The problem comes in when you are eating excessive sugar, because then you are placing an enormous burden on the pancreas. After a while, it is either no longer able to secrete enough insulin, or cells that usually respond to the hormone by taking sugar in and metabolizing it, no longer answer the door when insulin knocks. Either way, excess sugar remains in the blood.

Another problem: The pancreas can overreact to a sugar onslaught and produce *too much* insulin. Soon you have low blood sugar, or hypoglycemia. Combine these two problems and you've got an energy roller coaster. When your energy cycle plummets, you break for coffee and a doughnut for an energy boost. This works—very temporarily. Unfortunately, 20 minutes later the sugar is used up. This causes another energy withdrawal and the need for another sugar fix. This energy roller coaster is one you don't want to be on because, if uncorrected, a blood sugar imbalance may lead to more serious conditions, such as diabetes, heart disease, obesity, or candidiasis.

### 53 Eliminate bad food from your diet.

Getting healthy is not just a matter of putting good food into your body; it means taking the bad food out as well. This means you will have to change some learned habits that have been with you since childhood. I can hear you thinking, I can't give up my favorite snack foods; life would be so boring. Wrong!—on both counts. First, life wouldn't be boring because you'd be replacing your old snack foods with interesting new ones. Second, you *can* give up your snack foods if you do it gradually. From what I've observed, the most successful and lasting life changes are the ones that are part of a gradual process, one that begins with awareness.

## 54  Be alert to food allergies.

Even if you are eating well, allergies to common foods can compromise your health and vitality. Eating wheat, for example, may make you sleepy, and tomatoes may stiffen your joints. These are some common symptoms of allergy: fatigue, obesity, headaches, digestive symptoms, diminished concentration, nervousness, forgetfulness or memory lapses, hyperactivity and other behavior problems, learning disorders, inability to think clearly, a "spacey" sensation, skin problems, candida, and lower back pain. Any part of your body can become affected.

If you suspect you have an allergy problem, keeping a diary of what you eat can help you determine if this is the case, at least in regard to diet. Recording what you eat will help you to see patterns and make connections.

One effective way to keep a record is to divide a notebook page in half. Put the date on the top. On one side, note the time and what foods you ate. On the other side, record symptoms and the times they appear. To indicate severity, use one plus sign to indicate mild, two to indicate moderate, and three to indicate severe. After several days, you may begin to notice patterns.

What if your food diary entries lead you to suspect that you're allergic to a particular food? To test that idea, take a food challenge. What you do is eliminate the food from your diet for four days. On the fifth day, you eat that food alone. If you suspect wheat, for example, omit all forms of wheat for four days, and on the fifth day eat a bowl of cracked wheat made with just water. If you have a reaction to that food, it will probably show up right away or within two hours. (Other reactions do take longer; a trained physician can help here. Doctors of environmental medicine are particularly tuned in to dietary and other types of allergies.)

## 55 Put your foods on a four-day rotation.

If you want to minimize and prevent allergic reactions, you should get into the habit of following a four-day rotation diet. This isn't difficult or complicated; in fact there's just one thing to remember: Don't eat any potential allergen (allergy-causer) more than once every four days. For example, if your menu features brown rice on Monday, then the next time brown rice can appear is Friday. Peanuts, eaten Tuesday, return to your table no sooner than Saturday. (You can eat the rice, or the peanuts, more than just once on the days they are rotated into your diet. Just keep each portion moderate.)

Getting out of a diet rut and into rotational eating is good not just because it cuts down on allergic reactions; it also ensures that you eat a varied diet and thus consume a range of nutrients.

## 56 Cook.

Some people don't do it any more. They say they don't have time. Or that it's too much work. Or that going out is more fun.

Not true for excuses one and two, if you know some culinary strategies (see next entry). As for excuse three, I'll concede that going out can be fun, but it usually isn't fun for your body because of the make-up of the dishes you're served.

The truth is, there is nothing like a wholesome home-cooked meal. When you buy your own ingredients, you know exactly what goes into your food. Restaurants use salt and gravies to improve taste, but when you cook at home, you can make foods appetizing with less fattening ingredients. Another reason home is better is economy. Unless money is no object, you need to consider that when you dine out, you pay a lot for the stuff you don't eat, such as the service. What about the convenience of eating out? If you've prepared a few meal components ahead of time, or even if you've kept a well-stocked kitchen, eating at home can be quicker. You don't have to get ready to go out, and there's no travel time. Place some flowers on the table, dim the lights, and you've got ambiance as well. All of which is why I say, "There's no place like home."

### 57 Learn to cook—right now.

I've often said it isn't hard to cook. It's time to prove it. In just five steps, here's how to cook myriad nutritious, delicious, guest-impressive meals, with a minimum of fuss. You use a mix 'n' match approach, combining a grain base with a vegetable topping, adding protein complements and a raw salad if you wish. You don't need to slavishly follow specific recipes with this approach, which saves a lot of time and effort.

1. Cook your grain. Popular ones are rice and pasta. For rice, use brown. Boil 2 ⅓ cups water. Stir in 1 cup brown rice. Simmer, covered, for 30–50

minutes, depending on the brand. Add more water toward the end of cooking time if necessary.

For pasta, whole wheat is preferable to white. Boil a large pot of water. Add pasta; keep water at a boil for 5 to 13 minutes, depending on thickness and type of pasta, stirring from time to time. Taste pasta periodically, and when it has reached *al dente* stage, meaning that it's still got some firmness to it, drain. Toss pasta with a small amount of oil if you don't want it sticking together.

2. Meanwhile, prepare a mix of vegetables— organically grown ones, if possible—by stir frying until cooked but still firm, in a small amount of oil. (See next section for more on stir frying.) Some great ones to use: onions, carrots, peppers, mushrooms, zucchini, sugar snap peas, eggplant, green beans, broccoli, cauliflower (thin pieces), or whatever you have on hand. (Don't use potatoes; they're better baked.) Stir in desired seasoning—for example, tamari soy sauce for an Oriental-type dish, oregano for Italian. Use your imagination and experiment.

You can, alternatively, steam the vegetables, for a more lo-cal dish. Cover your steaming pot, keep the water line just below the veggies, and don't cook the things beyond minimum doneness. Add flavorings when steaming is done.

3. Combine your grain base and vegetables. To impress folks: Spread your rice or other grain base all around on a low, wide serving dish. Top with a vegetable mixture, spreading not quite to the edge of the dish, so that the grain shows at the edges. Garnish, depending on the dish, with celery or parsley flakes, other herbs, lemon wedges, or a good sprinkling of nuts, for added protein.

4. Other ways to add protein to your meal: Add fish or tofu to your stir fry. Add beans, such as

chickpeas or lentils, to your grain. Dried beans can be cooked in quantity, according to package directions, and then divided up for use in a few different meals. Two kinds of dried beans that cook quickly and do not require presoaking are lentils and split peas. You can also use canned beans for quick meals.

5. Feature a tossed salad in your meal. You can mix up a jumbo pot of washed, spun-dried, and cut-up fresh organic produce, and draw on it for several days' worth of meals.

### 58 Develop your skillet skills—stir fry.

Stir frying is healthier than deep frying because it's faster; thus, less oil is absorbed and fewer nutrients are lost.

The first step is choosing your skillet or wok. Ideally, it should be made of carbon steel, a thin metal that conducts heat quickly and evenly. However, any large frying pan will do. Carbon steel rusts easily, so you need to season it before its first use. This means filling the pan halfway with an inexpensive oil and heating until it smokes. After the pan begins to smoke, turn the heat off and allow the pan to sit overnight with hot oil in it. In the morning, pour off the oil and wipe the pan clean. This process need only be done once. Now you are ready for some enjoyable cooking.

The trick to stir frying is having all the ingredients prepared ahead of time and ready to go. Heat the oil until it's quite hot. (Make sure no water gets in the pan, as it will spatter.) Add ingredients and stir until cooked. If you are making a combination dish, add the longer-cooking foods first. Sometimes tougher vegetables, such as broccoli or carrots, are blanched first and then stir fried. You can also cover the pan and allow vegetables to cook in their own steam (over lower heat).

Have fun developing your own stir-fry combinations. Here's a recipe of mine for a combo you probably never would have thought of.

### STIR-FRY APPLES AND CELERY

*2 tablespoons unsalted butter*

*2 tablespoons sesame oil*

*1 tablespoon lemon juice*

*2 cups thinly sliced celery*

*2 medium apples, peeled, cored, and sliced thin*

*Salt*

*Pepper*

Heat butter and oil in a large skillet or wok. Stir in the lemon juice and celery; fry over high heat for 5 minutes, or until almost tender.

Add the apples. Continue cooking and stirring for 5 minutes or until tender.

Sprinkle with salt and pepper to taste.

SERVES 2 TO 3 AS AN ENTREE. CAN BE SERVED HOT OR COLD.

### 59 Bake more than cake.

You're probably familiar with baked fish, muffins, and breads, but less accustomed to baked vegetables, other than the standard baked potato. I recommend that you try baking all kinds of vegetables. Simply brush oil on the produce and place it in a baking pan. Sprinkle with herbs, if you wish. Then bake to produce a crispy snack or side dish that is less caloric than its fried counterpart.

Speaking of baking, I even bake spaghetti! Actually, I cook it on the stove first, but I have a baked spaghetti casserole that you might want to try because it's totally different, and great tasting.

## BAKED SPAGHETTI CASSEROLE

*6 ounces potato*
*6 ounces spaghetti, cooked*
*3 ounces tomato, chopped medium fine*
*4 ounces scallions, chopped medium fine*
*1 ½ ounces sesame seeds*
*1 ½ tablespoons sesame oil*
*¼ teaspoon thyme*
*4 teaspoons minced garlic*
*1 teaspoon salt*

Preheat oven to 400°. Lightly grease a 4x8-inch baking pan with small amount of sesame oil. Bake potato for 40 minutes. When cooled, cut into ½ -inch cubes. Lower heat to 375°. Combine all ingredients, transfer to baking pan, and bake for 15 minutes.

SERVES 2.

 **Control your cholesterol level intelligently.**

Even eliminating cholesterol-rich foods completely won't do it. You have to be a little more savvy about cutting your serum cholesterol level.

A key cholesterol-fighting tactic is to add more fiber-containing foods to your diet. You probably already know that a fiber-abundant diet lowers your risk of developing certain cancers. But fiber is important, too, in increasing the speed at which your body eliminates cholesterol. Pectin, found in apples, is especially good for this. Rolled oats, barley, and buckwheat are also valuable as cholesterol collectors. Try starting your day with these cereals, adding in apple pieces.

You should be aware that a small amount of polyunsaturated fats in the diet may lower serum cholesterol levels by 5 or 10 percent. Like roughage, they force cholesterol concentrations out of the blood. Linoleic acid, found in cold-pressed oils, fish (not shellfish), nuts, seeds, and nut butters, is especially good. I generally suggest lowering your fat intake to 15 percent of your dietary intake, and switching over to the unsaturated variety.

Vitamins and minerals play a role, too, in the cholesterol and heart-health picture. Are you deficient in vitamins that keep cholesterol levels under control? Niacin (vitamin $B_3$) is missing from most people's diets. You can find this valuable nutrient in salmon and tuna, and of course, a good B complex vitamin wouldn't hurt. One of wonderful vitamin C's many wonders is that it helps to lower cholesterol, so be sure to get at least 1 gram a day. Combine with lecithin and you dissolve arterial plaque. Include C's partner, the bioflavonoids, especially rutin and quercetin, and you get additional help. Vitamin E will help improve circulation to the heart.

As for minerals, studies reveal that chromium has cholesterol-lowering effects. Other important minerals for a healthy heart include calcium, magnesium, and zinc.

And don't forget herbs. To help the body use more cholesterol, eat more ginger and cayenne. Studies show that these herbs lower the liver's production of cholesterol and triglycerides. In addition, make sure to get plenty of garlic. Garlic lowers cholesterol and thins the blood, lowering your chances of dangerous blood clots. Raw garlic is most effective, but cooking with the herb also has a therapeutic effect. Deodorized capsules and pills are least effective, because they remove allicin, the smelly part of garlic that makes it most useful.

Lastly, avoid refined sugars, which lead to an unhealthy buildup of fats in your liver and tissues. They also lower your level of healthy high-density lipoproteins and increase the unwanted low-density ones. Replace refined foods with complex carbohydrates found in fruits, vegetables, and whole grains. Alcohol is high in refined sugar and should also be avoided.

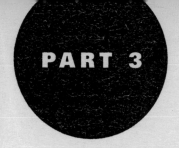

# PART 3

# LOSING WEIGHT AND LIKING IT

● ● ● ● ● ● ● ● ● ● ● ● ● ● ● ● ● ● ● ● ●

*So you want to lose weight. Great, because there's good news and there's better news. The good news, which you've probably already heard, is that you don't have to go on a specific, time-restricted, weight-loss diet, because these are obsolete. (They don't work, since the dieter always rebounds once the time is up.) The better news is that the smart-eating-for-the-rest-of-your-life plan that you do have to go on will make you feel wonderful, and help ward off disease. There's no downside here. So read on.*

**61 Go back to the very beginning (before the dawn of history!) to understand why we're overweight.**

Let's start with a prehistoric perspective on how fat forms and disappears. You still carry the fat-forming ability of your ancestors, the Neanderthals, and that ability was an efficient, handy thing to have—at the time. That's because, at the time, you didn't have supermarkets, three meals a day, and snacks any time you felt like it. You only had food when you hunted successfully, or came across a dead animal or some berries.

So whenever you found something edible, you considered yourself lucky, and you gorged. After all, you didn't have refrigerators either and there was no way to store what you found. Like a lion, you would eat until you could no longer move. After that you would just lay around for days, to conserve calories. Of course you would eventually have to start exercising again, to begin the search for more food. So you'd soon shed the extra fat.

Today, we're still really good at following this prehistoric pattern—the first three-quarters of it. That is, we're still good at gorging till we can't move. And at laying around a lot after that. And at putting on extra fat. The problem comes when we get to the part about eventually exercising to look for more food. We don't have to do that anymore; we just hop in the car and go to the store. Hence, a lot of people today have a lot of extra fat.

To determine whether you're one of them, don't just rely on your scale; take an impedance test. This is a simple, painless measure of your proportion of body fat, protein, lean muscle tissue, and water. The ideal percentage of fat for most men is in the low teens, and for women in the high teens.

But most people are 10 points above this level.

If you do need to reduce fat, remember that a sensible eating and exercise program is the only way to go.

### 62 Think about how you got to where you are today, both weight-wise and health-wise.

Specifically, think about the way family and cultural upbringing have shaped the way you've learned to eat. For instance, if you grew up in a household where the usual dinner consisted of hamburgers and fries or sending out for pizza, you probably continue to eat that way as an adult. You may also eat ice cream or candy to feel better if these foods were used to comfort you as a child. Or perhaps your parents equated "cleaning your plate" with being good. Unfortunately, the habits many of us learned as children are not the best for weight control, not to mention lifelong health.

It's hard to break away from the dietary patterns you learned in childhood, because there's more involved than just food; there's a whole overlay of emotions that can stop you from making changes. Plus there can be a whole set of relatives who take offense when you start to make changes! You don't want every family gathering to be a source of conflict. On the other hand, you don't want to sacrifice your health because others don't understand the changes you're making. So you may have to do some soul-searching before you can really launch into a new way of eating.

If you are ready to break away from traditional patterns and begin eating for weight control and maximum nutrition, you may wonder how to begin. First, you need to take a really good look at your present diet. In my opinion, keeping a food diary is the best way to do this.

### 63 Keep a food diary, and tell it the truth!

"Dear Diary, Today I ate a whole box of dough-nuts. . . "

Well, that's not *exactly* how you do it. What you do is simply keep a meal-by-meal record of every-thing you eat and drink over a period of several weeks. And a snack-by-snack record, too. Include amounts. By keeping a written record of what goes into your system—midnight refrigerator raids and all—you're taking the first step in honestly analyz-ing how you can improve your eating habits.

In case you're wondering, it's important that your food diary be an actual written record, and not just a list that you keep in your head. Mental food diaries are notoriously incomplete; it's easy to "for-get" large parts of your daily intake.

Once you've kept a food diary for a week or two, these are some questions you may begin to ask: Is my diet high in fats? Are the fats in my diet satu-rated? Unsaturated? Do I eat complex carbohydrates? Am I getting as many fruits and vegetables as I thought I did? Or am I eating mostly refined foods? Do I get most or all of my protein from animal prod-ucts? Am I eating too much of any particular food? Am I skipping breakfast? Your food diary will reveal all. And if you seek the help of a nutritionist or a nutritionally oriented health professional, which I do recommend, such a diary will be an invaluable aid.

Here's a fun idea. A year into your new, improved dietary regime, keep another food diary. Compare it with your first one. You'll get a sense of accomplishment similar to the sense of satisfaction you get from your new, improved body.

## 64 Take the first step to lose weight: detoxify.

Detoxification is vital for weight control. Your body doesn't work right if it's polluted. And if you are like most Americans, foods that pollute the body and undermine health are a way of life. Pizza, fried foods, and confections take center stage. Fresh fruit is not a priority. The only fresh vegetable you encounter on most days may be parsley, a garnish you toss aside. And take note: Even your "good" dietary habits may not be so great. The low-fat cookies you buy as a token of good intent are still refined carbohydrates with lots of sugar and chemical additives. And iceberg lettuce salads, heavily coated with sugary dressing and then festooned with oily croutons, hardly qualify as health food!

It all adds up to a nutritionally shortchanged lifestyle that deprives you of essential vitamins and minerals at the same time that it fills you with empty calories, and with chemicals. These poisons get into your fat and muscles and do nothing to help your body. On the contrary, they drain you of energy by disrupting normal biochemical processes. And one byproduct of a disrupted biochemistry is a slow metabolism, which is the process whereby your body burns food. When your body loses the wherewithal to burn food efficiently, your system gets out of balance, and you can gain a significant amount of weight.

All of which is why the first, and arguably the most important, step to getting in shape is detoxification. You've got to make a clean sweep so that you give your body a chance to rejuvenate and to function in a balanced way. This will allow the process of rebuilding to occur. Otherwise, you cannot benefit from any diet, no matter how good, because your body has to contend with too much interference from all the stuff that's clogging it up. Think of how much better you function at home once you've done a thorough spring cleaning and cleared out the clutter from your household. That's how much better your body's going to function once you've detoxified.

There are two main principles of detoxification. One is that you keep out the bad foods. Stay away from foods that congest your system, such as fats, refined foods, and chemical additives. Reduce meat and dairy, as they create mucus and clog you up. Also beware of foods that tend to stimulate the appetite, such as hot spices, and salted, pickled, fried, and sugary foods.

In general, also stay away from diuretics, and from high-protein diets. Consult a holistically oriented doctor knowledgeable in nutrition for advice on a detoxification eating plan that's right for you.

The second thing you absolutely must do to detoxify is exercise. Even if you think you lack the energy, get yourself moving daily. Sweating means that you are detoxifying through your skin. And exercise lowers your setpoint, your internal weight-regulating mechanism.

## 65 To help with detoxification, take extra vitamin C.

Use vitamin C in the form of sodium ascorbate to promote detoxification and to lessen uncomfortable symptoms that accompany a withdrawal from addictive substances, allergy-producing foods, and toxic chemicals. You can work with a physician who administers vitamin C intravenously, or take bowel-tolerance doses on your own. This means taking a teaspoon of sodium ascorbate every three to four hours to the point of diarrhea, and then backing off to just slightly below that dosage. This may sound awful, but it's actually simple to do, and it lets you know the exact amount you need to detoxify your system and reduce unpleasant symptoms.

(In case you haven't heard, vitamin C does a whole lot more than detoxify. It's an antiaging, antidisease nutrient that performs a wide variety of tasks, from synthesizing collagen, which forms the body's connective tissue, to combating stress. We'll be looking at it more closely in the next section.)

**66** **Use fiber to make a clean sweep.**

Eating high-fiber foods is essential for the detox process. Of course it's a good idea for the rest of your life, too.

In case you're confused about fiber, here's what you have to know. First, here's what has *no* fiber: meat, dairy products, and highly processed foods. Fiber's found everywhere else, that is to say, in fruits, vegetables, grains, nuts, and seeds. Just remember—it's a plant thing. So if you eat a wide variety of plant foods in their natural, unrefined form, you'll get soluble and insoluble fiber, both of which are good for you. (Insoluble has a mechanical scrubbing action, and soluble lowers cholesterol.) Some super sources of fiber: root vegetables, such as carrots; legumes, such as lentils, beans, and peas—especially sprouts made from these; whole-grain cereals; citrus fruits.

A tasty vehicle for dietary fiber is the muffin; unfortunately, most commercially produced muffins contain a lot of fat, so you're not getting the "health food" you think you are. Here's a favorite high-fiber muffin recipe of mine that's truly healthful. By the way, muffins are quick and so easy to make—all you need to mix them up is a bowl and a spoon.

**GARY'S MAGIC MUFFINS**

1 cup whole wheat flour
2 cups bran
½ cup safflower oil
⅓ cup honey
⅔ cup molasses
1 cup water
1 teaspoon vanilla
¼ teaspoon allspice
¼ teaspoon nutmeg
2 bananas, mashed
½ cup raisins
¼ cup chopped pecans
1 teaspoon salt

Preheat oven to 350°. Combine all ingredients in a mixing bowl; mix well until blended. Pour the batter into a greased muffin tin until each cup is two-thirds full. Bake for 30–45 minutes, until the tops are golden brown.

MAKES 12 LARGE MUFFINS, OR MORE SMALL ONES.

**67 Use herbs to cleanse your body.**

Different herbs will help you to cleanse specific body systems:

**CLEANSING HERBS: WHERE THEY WORK**

| | |
|---|---|
| Liver | Milk thistle, licorice root, and Siberian ginseng pep up a sluggish liver. Safe for short-term use. |
| Bowels | Dandelion root and yellow dock are gentle cleansers. |
| Kidneys | Dandelion leaf is a natural diuretic. |
| Skin | Nettle and burdock help toxins leave the skin. Echinacea helps get rid of eczema, acne, and boils. |
| Lungs | Elecampane helps smokers clear lungs. Add mullein flowers to hot water and breathe in the vapors. |

## CLEANSING HERBS: WHERE THEY WORK (*cont.*)

| | |
|---|---|
| Immune system | Echinacea and goldenseal at the first sign of a cold often nip it in the bud. Use only for a few days. For long-term benefit, try garlic. |

Herbs are even good at helping you reduce fat and appetite. Try chickweed, burdock root, or nettle tea between meals.

### 68 Now, rebuild your body, using only the best materials.

Once you cleanse your system, rebuilding is a simple process. Just put in the good stuff—only what you need, now—and let your body do the rest. It will naturally seek a thinner, healthier you without a whole lot of interference on your part. As a result, you'll look, feel, think, and act better.

The basic advice on rebuilding for weight control is to follow a diet that is high in complex carbohydrates and low in protein and fat. Be sure to include plenty of salads and steamed cruciferous vegetables, such as broccoli, cauliflower, brussels sprouts, and cabbage, on a daily basis. Other good foods include asparagus, lemons, green leafy vegetables, carrots, cantaloupe, celery, tomatoes, melons, berries, plums, sesame seeds, and garlic.

Plants from the sea—these include kombu, wakame, hijiki, nori, agar, kuzu, kelp, algin, sea palm, and dulse—will supply you with calcium, iodine, and many important trace minerals lacking in our soil today. Iodine plays a major role in managing your body's metabolic speed, so it may be especially important in helping you to lose weight.

Make sure to include starchy high-fiber foods, such as potatoes, yams, squash, and whole-grain pastas. These foods are digested rather slowly, which allows you to benefit energy-wise from their sugars for up to several hours. While many dieters avoid starches, believing that these foods are fattening, they're wrong. In truth, starchy foods are low in calories; it's the add-ons, such as butter and sour cream, that are the problem. Plus starches are rich in minerals and vitamins; a potato, for example, has as much vitamin C as an orange.

Note that when you eat this way—concentrating on complex carbohydrates and holding down the fats—you don't have to go on a "diet" diet, the kind where you slavishly weigh every bit of food and are restricted to mere morsels at each meal. That's the discredited kind of reducing regimen that works initially (at the price of a very bad mood!) but then fails you big-time when you go off it, because the scale zooms up like pounds were going out of style. No, this eating plan is for the rest of your life. You may lose weight more slowly with this diet than with the one-and-a-half-lettuce-leaves-for-lunch type, but the weight you lose will be permanently off, and you'll feel so much better, both mentally and physically, and both now and in the long run.

## 69 Eat more beans and legumes.

Eating more beans and legumes as your main source of protein will help you to trim down. These foods are excellent sources of vitamins and minerals, and their high fiber content fills you up more quickly than animal proteins do. Since your stomach feels satisfied sooner, you eat less. Voilà! Weight loss!

Have you had trouble with bean digestion? Learning how to cook beans properly can avoid embarrassing gas attacks. Before cooking, soak beans overnight. Then boil them for one or two hours. That removes most gas-producing properties.

Also, don't eat fruit or sugary foods with a bean meal.

Note that beans expand a lot when you cook them, so start with about one part beans to four parts water (or five, if you're making a soup). Alternatively, you can used canned beans, but they're not going to taste as good.

Now let's look at some specific legumes. Chickpeas, also known as garbanzos, are extremely versatile; they can be roasted as well as boiled, and ground up into bean pates or that Middle Eastern favorite, hummus. Stirred into rice or other grain dishes, they provide a delicate flavor complement. Chickpeas are high in calcium, iron, potassium, and B vitamins, as well as protein.

Kidney beans, the basis of delicious chilis, will cook in about an hour, after soaking.

In the Caribbean, Mexico, and parts of the American Southwest, black beans, and the closely related turtle beans, have been longtime staples. They make a delicious soup. Also favored in the Southwest are pinto beans, which are tasty in baked casseroles.

If you are short on time, lentils, navy beans, split peas, and black-eyed peas all cook in an hour or less and require no presoaking.

Mung beans make superb sprouts rich in vitamins A and C, as well as calcium, phosphorus, and iron.

Did you know that peanuts are a legume? They are, and peanut butter—pure and unadulterated, please—makes a good protein source. Don't go too crazy over this American favorite, though, because it has a high fat content.

Finally, there's that most nutritious of legumes, the soybean. Soybeans provide high-quality protein in a form that's better for your body than meat. The beans are less expensive than meat, too, and can be made into all sorts of foods, including soy flour, flakes, granules, and grits, as well as sprouts, dry-roasted snacks, miso, tempeh, and tofu.

Never tried tofu? Here's a superquick way that I like to use it.

**TANTALIZING TOFU**

>  6 ounces tofu, cut into bite-size pieces
>  6 ounces broccoli, cut into bite-size pieces
>  3 ounces turnip greens, coarsely chopped
>  1 ½ ounces walnuts, chopped
>  ½ teaspoon basil
>  ½ teaspoon salt
>  2 tablespoons soy oil
>  3 ounces romaine lettuce

Sauté all ingredients, except for the lettuce, in soy oil for 3 to 4 minutes. Arrange on a bed of lettuce.

SERVES 2.

## 70 Make soup.

Soup, with its filling water base, is a wonderful weight-loss food. Don't rely on canned soups, though; they tend to be very salty, and don't taste all that fresh—because they're not. That's why I believe you should make your own.

And listen—don't make the mistake of believing in the soup-cookery mystique. What I mean is, some people have the idea that cooking soup is really hard. Well, maybe it was in pioneer days, when you had to kill the animal you were making the soup out of, and then cook it in the fireplace. But we're not using animal foods, remember? And I assume you have a stove. So forget your doubts and try it! This recipe is easy, and unbeatably good.

## LENTIL BARLEY SOUP

*2 tablespoons safflower oil*
*2 cups lentils*
*1 cup barley*
*1 cup chopped onions*
*6–8 cups water*
*1 cup sliced celery*
*½ cup sliced carrots*
*½ teaspoon tarragon, or to taste*
*Salt to taste*
*Pepper to taste*

In a large saucepan, heat the oil and sauté the lentils, barley, and onion until the onion is translucent, about 5 minutes.

Add the water. Bring the mixture to a boil and then reduce the flame. Simmer for about 20 minutes or until the barley is tender.

Add the celery and carrots. Season to taste and cook for another 10 minutes or until the carrots are done.

SERVES 6.

## 71 Deep-six the deep-fried!

It's obvious from a dieting standpoint that eating french fries, onion rings, and doughnuts is an unwise choice calorie-wise, but you may not know just how unhealthful these foods are. They're prepared in fatty oils that have been heated to high temperatures. This alters the chemical structure of oils and makes it more difficult for the body's enzymes to break them down. Therefore, your body must work harder and longer just to make use of the stuff.

As a result, other parts of your body must sacrifice energy toward digestion, so you feel tired, listless, and rundown. This also has an irritating effect on your stomach and intestines, and can ultimately lead to serious problems such as colitis, spastic colon, or irritable bowel syndrome.

Eating well is more than what you eat, then. It's how you prepare foods. Potatoes, for instance, are good for you, but once fried, they absorb oils that are not worth it as far as your system is concerned. Bottom line, stay away from deep-fried foods.

While we're on the subject of potatoes, if you yourself are the couch type, the problem of excess fat in your diet is going to be compounded. That's because if you don't exercise, the fat you eat tends to take the place of the muscles that you don't use. As a result, you lose strength, endurance, and stamina, and are more prone to disease and injury. This also means that if you start to exercise, it will be far more difficult to get going. Not only will you need to build muscle—but you'll need to get rid of the fat that's in its place.

### 72 If you shouldn't eat it, don't keep it! (Don't even *read* about it!)

Are you really serious about losing weight and eating more healthfully? Then it's time to play out-with-the-old, in-with-the-new.

To prevent compulsive eating at home, keep only the good foods around. Take an inventory of your cabinets, refrigerator, and freezer. Clean them out and put back only those foods are going to have a positive impact on your health. Everything else can be given away or thrown away. Canned goods, for instance, can be donated to a food drive. Cookbooks that have sentimental value but are no longer useful can be stored away with old family pictures. Just making a clean sweep like this will make you feel lighter right away.

A note concerning cookbooks: Have you checked out the cooking sections of your local bookstores lately? They're expanding like crazy, with lots of wonderful new books on vegetarian

**SUPERCHARGE YOUR HEALTH!**

and low-fat cooking. And don't pass by the ethnic cookbooks, especially those featuring Oriental and Mexican cuisines, where plant foods have long been a culinary mainstay.

### 73 Eliminate excuses.

Excuses are for children. They're even cute: *The dog ate my homework.* But for adults on a fitness or weight loss regimen? *The dog ate my salad, so I had to eat three candy bars instead?* No, that doesn't quite cut it.

Yet we adults come up with so many excuses.

*I know I should exercise, but there are too many other things to do.*

*I had to order that rich dessert so that my friends wouldn't feel bad about doing the same.*

*I do usually walk three miles a day—unless it's cold, hot, windy, or wet out, or I get involved in a long phone call.*

You can make excuses. Or you can make yourself fit. You can't do both.

### 74 Look at *how* you eat.

While it's important to look at *what* you eat, I'm always reminding people that it is equally important to look at *the way* you eat. For instance, do you chew once or twice and then bolt the food down with water? Or do you take the time to aid digestion by chewing properly? Do you eat your food crisp, fried, supersalty, or sweet? Are you relaxed when you eat, or are you nervous? Must you always have the television or radio on? Is mealtime family friction time? These factors all set the stage for how your body copes with what you take in.

If you have a weight problem, pay particular attention to these questions about eating habits: Do you eat as an accompaniment to TV watching or reading? If so, your portion control may be way out of whack, or nonexistent. Do you forget to chew? If so, you're not only hindering digestion, you're eating too quickly for your body to register a feeling of fullness before it's too late. Do you use fattening foods as rewards, celebration centerpieces, or consolation prizes? Recipes for disaster, all.

I consider all of these bad habits to be examples of "mindless" eating. Be *mindful* of how you eat. Plan out your meal and snack times, not just as to food selections, but in terms of the experience of each. It will make a big difference in how you feel and look.

## 75 Take eating disorders seriously.

Anorexia nervosa and bulimia are sweeping our thinness-obsessed society, and eating disorders are especially prevalent among young women, who grow up facing a constant barrage of unrealistic skinnier-than-thou images. Anorexic individuals self-starve, while bulimics eat large quantities of food and then purge themselves to avoid weight gain. Both conditions are related to deep-rooted psychological problems, but their consequences go far beyond the psychological: Complete bodily breakdown and even death can result from these disorders.

If you are suffering from an eating disorder, it is imperative to seek professional help. Treatment should combine psychological approaches with nutrition. Zinc, in particular, may be needed. Zinc sulfate solution, a liquid form of the mineral, is absorbed most easily.

## 76 Know this: Exercise is more important than dieting for weight management.

Surprised? Think about it a moment. If dieting alone worked, then why is the market always crowded with so many new diet programs?

Most diets are based on the following premise: Since 3500 kilocalories equal 1 pound, you gain a pound whenever you exceed your intake by that amount, and you lose a pound whenever you take in that much less. Moreover, the effect is cumulative. Eating one extra slice of bread a day equals 490 extra calories a week, and 10 extra pounds a year.

Sound logical? Yes. But the body doesn't work this way. Otherwise, there wouldn't be thin people who eat all day long, and overweight people who eat far less. This calorie counting theory fails to take into account the body's setpoint mechanism, and the vital role that exercise plays.

## 77 Be aware of the setpoint setup.

Have you ever dieted and lost weight briefly, only to see the pounds quickly return? What happened was you were being set up for weight-loss failure by your setpoint. You see, human beings have a built-in mechanism, known as a setpoint, that is designed to keep weight consistent. Scientists tell us that the setpoint was useful for primitive man, who needed such a device to prevent starvation. Since food was not always available, our ancestors would alternate between gluttony and fasting. To keep from starving, the body learned to store food as fat when a lot was eaten, and to burn it slowly when none was there.

Today, our bodies still work the same way. That's why going on a starvation diet, or even just eating less than usual, causes us to conserve energy and store fat. It's a protective mechanism. The body will strive to store any food that it gets until it reaches a predetermined setpoint, that is, a level of fat it considers necessary for its functioning.

You can look at your *setpoint* as a sort of body-weight thermostat. If a thermostat is set at 70 degrees, any temperature lower than that activates the furnace to raise the room temperature. Similarly, if your body's setpoint is at 165 pounds, any weight lower than that will tell the body it needs to store more fat. Our setpoint is regulated by a center in the brain known as the hypothalamus, which regulates many bodily functions, such as temperature, sleep, and appetite.

One way the setpoint gets you to keep your weight up is to increase your appetite. That's why dieters feel excessively hungry until they get back to their previous weight. The setpoint is why, with dieting, *whatever goes down, must come up* seems to be the unfortunate rule of thumb, and why we have the phenomenon of the yo-yo syndrome, with dieters losing weight and regaining it over and over again.

## 78 Understand the setpoint/aerobics connection.

Just as not every thermostat is set at 68 degrees, people have different setpoints, with genetics playing a role in this. Thin people seem to be just naturally better at turning food into energy, and overweight people at storing it. If storing food as fat comes a little too naturally to you, you've got to find a way to reset your inner regulatory mechanism.

But how the heck do you reset that thing? It's easy to reset the thermostat on your wall; all it takes is the turn of a dial. But what do you do to reset your inner setpoint—go into your brain and give your hypothalamus a twist? I don't know whether that's doable, but personally, I'd find that approach a bit invasive. Especially considering that there's a much less messy way!

You see, you can change your inner thermostat from fat to fit through steady aerobic exercise. A routine of 20 to 30 minutes, performed within your target heart rate three to five times a week, is the recommended way to go. Choose running, power walking, bicycling, rowing, or any one of various other aerobic activities. Better yet, choose more than one. (See Part 5, on exercise.) The point is that an aerobics routine is not just a frill; it's the key to your success in losing weight. Just as important, it will improve the functioning of your heart and lungs.

Always remember that the cumulative effect of exercising is what counts, not any one session. The whole program allows your body to produce more muscle than fat. Over time, your body's chemistry changes so that your metabolism improves, and you burn calories more efficiently. Eventually, your setpoint lowers, and you burn calories faster even after your exercise period ends.

## 79 To lose those last few stubborn pounds. . . add some action.

Sometimes the last few nagging pounds are the hardest to get rid of. Even though you've been eating right and exercising, you seem to have reached your limit. A prime way to get over this weight loss hump is to add some more action to your life. You may not be exercising as much as your body needs, so start exerting more energy. A little extra energy spent, day after day, can have a big payoff. So walk up the stairs instead of relying on elevators and escalators. Walk farther and for longer periods of time; go the extra mile and you'll lose the extra pound. Take bike rides regularly.

This might be the perfect time to join a jogging, cycling, or hiking club. You'll be around people who will encourage your efforts, making adding that bit of extra action to your life easy, and fun!

### 80 Don't let the scale scare you.

Muscle weighs more than fat. So as you're struggling to reach a weight goal, don't be upset if a little fat turns to muscle and increases your weight rather than decreases it. If this has happened, put your scale away for awhile; it will only discourage you. A tape measure and the fit of your clothes will show you the extent of the progress that is being made. Ultimately, continued aerobic exercise combined with your reformed eating habits will result in weight loss.

### 81 Eat less.

This is a real no-brainer, isn't it? Still, it's worth asking yourself whether the reason you've still got those five or ten extra pounds is simply that you're eating too much. Granted, when you're close to your desired weight, you sometimes become less motivated to reach the finish line. Most Americans carry some extra poundage, and being a little overweight doesn't carry the social stigma that obesity does. So it's easy to forget about your original weight goal and fool yourself into thinking that a piece of cake or some chips won't hurt. Yet wouldn't it be nice to actually hit that target weight right on the bull's-eye?

You can do it. Cut portion sizes. Don't help

yourself to seconds. Forego desserts. All these little steps will soon add up, or rather, subtract, in the case of your weight!

## 82  Be party-ready.

Something that might make the difference in terms of weight loss is planning a strategy for when you socialize. Social activities usually center around food. Friends dine out at restaurants and families feast at home. At a party, well-meaning hosts say, "Just one won't hurt," or tell you, "You're thin enough." You need a way to counter these pressures.

This is not to say that you should be unsociable. It just means that you may need to take extra precautions when you are in the company of others. Learn a few little tricks.

**SIX PARTY TRICKS**
1. Before going to a party, eat a healthful mini-meal at home so that you are less tempted to snack.
2. When you go out with friends, take wholesome snacks along. As they stuff themselves with cookies, pizza, and sodas, satisfy your own hunger with grapes, a banana, or an apple.
3. Drinking plenty of pure water will help keep cravings away.
4. When you dine out, order sensibly. You'll find that the plain, lower-calorie food, a few minutes after it's eaten, is just as satisfying as the calorie-laden creamy dish. By the way, anything on the menu can be served without its accompanying sauce, or with the sauce on the side, if you ask.
5. If you're the host, center entertainment around interests other than eating. For example, have a movie or theater party, a fall foliage walk, a book discussion evening, or a tennis or badminton after-

noon. You may think a new entertainment style would be hard to institute if you've been entertaining the same group the same way for many years. It's not as hard as you think, though; your friends will probably welcome the change of pace.

6. Lastly, here's a friend-keeping tip. If you're at a party or other gathering and eating differently from everyone else, don't talk about it unless you're asked. When you are, it's fine to explain your eating style to those who are genuinely curious. Cut off conflict-seekers, though; you're at a party to have fun, not to fight.

## 83 Learn to love yourself more.

Think about this: Do you use food as a way of punishing yourself? It's possible that, secretly, you may be eating because you do not feel you deserve to be healthy, happy, popular, or pretty. You also may be afraid of losing friends once your self-image changes. Overeating just enough to keep you from attaining your ideal weight keeps your life from changing.

Analyze what is bothering you; keeping a journal, as we've already discussed, can help you do this. Then, take steps to eliminate the problem. Get professional help, if you need it. Also, you might try using self-affirmations, positive statements you make to yourself that focus your mind in a better direction. This sounds simplistic, but a lot of people report that using the technique makes a difference. You say to yourself, for example:

*I'm allowed to look great.*

*I can attract admiring looks without feeling guilty about it.*

*It's my right to feel fantastic.*

*Eating well will help me make the most of my life, so of course I'm going to do that!*

*I'll be at my target weight in a month, because I deserve to be.*

*I've learned how to do it; now I'm going to.*

*There's no one stopping me but me, only I ain't doin' that no more!*

(Use bad grammar in self-affirmations, by all means; it can help!)

### 84 Be realistic about your weight.

Let's face it. Every woman just isn't meant to look like a stick-thin model. Even most stick-thin models aren't meant to look that way! The media sell us images that are less than authentic.

Our genetic makeup determines what our minimum weight should be. Losing any more is unhealthy. If your weight stabilizes at a point higher than your fantasy weight, ask yourself whether perhaps this is the weight you were naturally meant to be. If so, enjoy being who you naturally are.

And another word to the wise, and realistic, both women and men. As we've said before, muscle weighs more than fat. So you can be a muscular, optimally trim individual and be "overweight" on the charts. Conversely, your pound count can fit right in there on the charts, while you are actually overfat. An impedance test will tell, where the charts and your scale may not. So factor all this in when evaluating your progress.

### 85 Think before you eat—and before you don't!

Get into the habit of keeping your mind in gear vis-à-vis what goes into your mouth. This doesn't mean become obsessed. What it means is, think about what your body really needs at several points during a typical day—e.g., before you pop something into your mouth, during the course of a meal, and even when you're not eating. That way, you'll be less likely to eat beyond what you need to satisfy your hunger. You'll also be less likely to ignore hunger, which is important, too, because if you neglect the urge to eat, your appetite thermostat will eventually overpower you and cause you to binge. If you eat too much, you may raise your setpoint and gain weight.

By paying attention to your hunger, you may find that you need to eat several small meals each day, or that you can easily eat less overall, or that there's one particular time of day when social cues overwhelm bodily cues as to how much to eat. By being mentally in touch with your need for food, you'll be less likely to either overeat or starve yourself; you will be on the right track.

Just keep to your program of a good diet and regular exercise and, in time, you will look and feel like a new person. Don't expect results to appear all at once, but know that once they appear, they'll be here to stay.

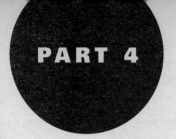

# PART 4

# VITAMINS, MINERALS, AND MORE

• • • • • • • • • • • • • • • • • • • •

*We've looked at how to eat, what to eat, and what not to eat. Let's delve into nutrition a little deeper and look at what's in the food we eat. Specifically, what are the vitamins, minerals, and enzymes that keep our bodies functioning at their best?*

## 86 Get enthused about vitamins and minerals.

Vitamins and minerals. Borrr-ing! You've been hearing about the darned things since you were a kid. But here's what's new about vitamins and minerals: improve your understanding of them, and optimize your intake, and you could be *feeling* like a kid again!

You see, vitamins aren't just for preventing deficiency diseases with weird names anymore. We now know that people can improve the way they feel and function by getting the right amounts of these vital substances. What's more, we can prevent major degenerative diseases, like cancer, by making wise use of what researchers have learned about vitamins recently. So it really pays to dip back into the subject of these nutrients and ask questions like, what do they do for us and where do we get them?

A first question might be, why are vitamins vital? No, you don't need vitamins as building blocks for your body—that's protein. But you do need them to *help* in the body-building process, and to make your bodily and mental functioning the best it can be. They're enablers.

More specifically, a vitamin is a natural organic compound that's needed, in small quantities, for the body to function normally. (Organic, here, means plant- or animal-based, or carbon-containing. So vitamins come from plant or animal sources, although they can be synthesized chemically as well.) In recent years, vitamins have been used therapeutically in the treatment and prevention of various conditions.

How do minerals differ? Vitamins are organic, but minerals, by contrast, are inorganic. A mineral is an element that the body needs in small amounts to function properly. The saying that good things come in small packages is applicable to minerals: While these substances comprise only 4 percent of your body weight, they are vital components of health.

### 87 Consider why you might need nutritional supplements.

You could be eating what appears to be the best diet in the world and still need to take supplemental nutrients. Why? Well, one very important reason is that food isn't what it used to be.

The problem is the soil. You may have a beautiful salad in front of you, but if the lettuce, carrots, and tomatoes in it were grown in soil that's been depleted of minerals, that salad's not quite the nutritional bonanza that it should be. And sadly, soil depleted of minerals is typical of American agribusiness. The practice of monoculture—planting the same crop on a piece of land over and over again—may be cheap and convenient, but it's not good for the soil. The same goes for the use of pesticides and artificial fertilizers. By contrast, practices that *are* good for the soil—crop rotation; the planting of winter, or cover crops; the use of manure for fertilizer; pesticide-free farming; and the maintaining of treed areas as windbreaks to prevent soil erosion—are more costly to large, bottom-line-oriented farming companies and therefore used less. Unfortunately, the American public pays a price in terms of diminished food quality.

Another reason you may need supplements is the health assaults we endure in modern society. We live with all types of pollution, from the kinds we can smell and taste, like air and water pollution, to the kinds we can't sense but are nevertheless there, i.e., the electromagnetic fields emanating from innumerable devices around us. All of this is not to scare you, but simply to explain why a health boost in the form of some extra nutrients might be in order.

## 88 Don't just go out and buy every supplement in the store—learn about your body first.

Anyone interested in optimizing health and energy should know what all the major nutrients do for the body. In fact, I'd go as far as to say that you're just not an educated person if you don't. But knowing about all the nutrients' benefits doesn't mean that you should be *taking* them all, as supplements. So after you read up on vitamins and minerals, please don't jump up and convert your kitchen cabinet into an extension of the local pharmacy. Instead, find out about your own unique needs by visiting a nutritionally oriented doctor and getting some tests done.

The following tests can help you and your doctor get a picture of where you stand, both nutritionally and in relation to other vital health concerns. You probably won't need them all; a physician will help you determine which are relevant to you. Once the results are in, you'll be in a position to plan, with the doctor's guidance, an intelligent diet and supplementation program.

**CLASSIC BLOOD TEST (SMA–24).** This test provides you and your doctor with a lot of important information. It tells you whether your blood is acid or too alkaline and whether your uric acid, calcium, and cholesterol levels are in balance. It also helps you to see if vitamin and mineral levels are low and, if so, how much supplementation is needed. In addition, it lets you see whether the nutrients in your food are properly absorbed.

This last question is too often overlooked. People think that the most important factor in nutrition is how many vitamins and minerals they are taking in. This is not correct, because you can be eating the best diet in the world, but it will do you no good if you are not properly metabolizing, that is, breaking down and using, the nutrients in your food. The fact is that detecting and correcting problems of metabolism is vital; it can prevent all sorts of physical and mental problems.

**GLUCOSE TOLERANCE TEST (GTT).** This test measures blood levels of glucose, which is the sugar that the body uses. When glucose is too high or too low, you feel lethargic, dizzy, or irritable. The GTT is a simple, inexpensive test that helps you see if blood sugar disturbances are altering your mood and lowering your energy level.

**COMPLETE BLOOD COUNT (CBC).** The CBC looks at red and white blood cells. White blood cells are the body's soldiers. A high count usually means that the internal army is attempting to fight off an infection, while a low blood count may indicate that there are not enough soldiers around and immunity is down. When red blood cells are too small, this indicates an iron deficiency. The body doesn't have enough iron or isn't properly handling the iron that it does have. If red blood cells are too large, there is probably a vitamin $B_{12}$ deficiency.

**VIRAL TITER.** This test measures immunoglobulin-G (IgG) and immunoglobulin-M (IgM). The IgG measure tells whether you were at one time infected with a virus or bacterium, while the IgM measure lets you know whether you are currently infected, to what degree you are infected, and what this infection might be doing to your system.

**AMINO ACID PANEL.** Amino acids are essential for good mood and overall health. Twenty-two amino acids and their metabolic breakdown products can be measured, and looking at their patterns can help physicians diagnose and treat a variety of physical and mental problems.

**THYROID FUNCTIONING TEST.** This test is important because a low thyroid level is a common cause of depression. Chronic fatigue may also be caused by a malfunctioning thyroid gland.

**HAIR ANALYSIS.** The best way to screen for heavy metals—such as mercury, lead, arsenic, aluminum, cadmium, and nickel—is hair analysis. Since hair growth is slow, a short strand will reflect the mineral status of the body over a period of months. If you receive a dental amalgam filling, for example, you can see an initial rise of mercury registered in the hair. In addition, a hair analysis will let you know if your body is not absorbing minerals efficiently, and if an imbalance is occurring due to a lack of calcium, magnesium, zinc, manganese, chromium, or some other mineral.

**TESTING FOR CHEMICAL SENSITIVITIES.** These tests tell you whether you are sensitive to major solvents and other chemicals found in the environment.

**IgG4 AND IgE TESTS.** These test for allergies to different foods, chemicals, and inhalants by identifying antibody responses in the blood.

**IMPEDANCE TEST.** This measures your percentage of body fat; as we've mentioned, it's better than the scale in determining whether you've accumulated too much fat.

89 **See all that C can do for you.**

Vitamin C is a water-soluble nutrient that has grown in popularity since word got out that it can prevent or stop a cold. While it is indispensable for this purpose, C is remarkable in other ways as well. In fact, I'd call it the superstar of the nutrients, and here's why.

First, this antioxidant works ceaselessly to strengthen the immune system. A strong immune system allows you to fight off colds and flus and other types of infections. It also helps you recover from injuries faster, and to get relief from allergies.

In addition, vitamin C helps keep cholesterol levels where they ought to be, protects against heart disease and cancer, builds strong bones and teeth, maintains mental health, and builds collagen, the "cement" that holds your tissues together.

Vitamin C is also a powerful detoxifier that plays a major role in any holistic program designed to treat mental illness, cancer, AIDS, chronic fatigue syndrome, emotional disturbances, drug addiction, or alcoholism. For serious conditions, megadoses (10 grams or more) of vitamin C are given intravenously or orally to neutralize destructive free radicals, get rid of toxic material, and stimulate the immune system.

### What happens if you don't get enough vitamin C?

The other name for vitamin C, ascorbic acid, comes from the Latin root, "a," *without*, and "scorbutus," *scurvy*. Scurvy, a condition marked by bleeding gums and bruised skin, plagued sailors hundreds of years ago, before a connection was made between the disease and a lack of vitamin C. Lemons and limes, which contain the vitamin, were added to ships' cargoes and the condition disappeared.

### Where can you get it?

Vitamin C is contained in fresh fruits and vegetables, particularly oranges, grapefruits, lemons, limes, tangerines, papaya, strawberries, cantaloupe, tomatoes, broccoli, red and green sweet peppers, potatoes, lettuce, and other leafy vegetables.

Note that to prevent vitamin C loss, you should store your foods in a cool place, and if you cook them, drink or re-utilize the cooking water. Processing and food shipping also zap vitamin C from foods, so if you can eat locally grown fresh produce, that's the way to go.

## How much should you take?

Since extra vitamin C is superprotective and nontoxic, it's a good idea to take a supplement, no matter how healthy you are. Vitamin C works especially well when combined with bioflavonoids, and many formulas combine the two.

According to official sources, the minimum daily requirement of vitamin C is 60 mg daily for the average adult. In my opinion, this is way too small an amount. For optimal health, nutritionists now recommend at least 500 to 1,000 mg (or 1 gram) daily. And if you are suffering from a serious disease such as cancer, a doctor who follows a nutritional approach may recommend bowel-tolerance doses, or administer 10 or more grams of C intravenously. This may sound excessive, but when you are sick your body needs more C and welcomes it. Anything extra leaves the system.

While most people experience no side effects from large doses of vitamin C, some do. This may be from taking it on an empty stomach, or from a supplement that uses an additive, flavoring, or chemical agent in its processing. A solution may be to take calcium ascorbate, a mild calcium compound that supplies you with the benefits of vitamin C and calcium. If that doesn't work, try stirring ⅙ teaspoon of pure vitamin C powder into room-temperature fruit or vegetable juice, and sipping it slowly after meals and before going to sleep. This method is particularly good if you have an ulcer or other stomach problems.

## 90 Boost C's benefits with bioflavonoids.

Bioflavonoids, or vitamin P, refer to a group of water-soluble substances that exist in nature wherever vitamin C is found. Like Batman and Robin, bioflavonoids and C work as a team to defend cells against dangerous elements. The vitaminlike qualities of bioflavonoids, i.e., their ability to facilitate cell function, is the reason scientists have given this group the honorary title of vitamin P.

When vitamin C is on patrol against bacteria and viruses, vitamin P is right alongside it. C takes care of the larger blood vessels, while P concentrates on smaller capillaries. It also helps C manufacture collagen and chelate (bind) harmful heavy metals, and then sweep them out of the body. The two nutrients work synergistically; that is, neither works as well alone as it does with the other.

Bioflavonoids aid in capillary care by allowing more life-sustaining nutrients to enter cells, and more waste products to leave. They are invaluable for anyone suffering from high blood pressure, strokes, atherosclerosis, blood flow and clotting disorders, and other disorders as well. Of course, they should ideally be taken before any sign of disease to maintain good health.

### What happens if you don't get enough vitamin P?

Too little vitamin P can lead to bleeding gums and easily bruised skin, the same symptoms that signal a vitamin C deficiency.

### Where can you get vitamin P?

Excellent sources of bioflavonoids are grapes, rosehips, prunes, oranges, lemon juice, cherries, black currants, plums, parsley, grapefruit, cabbage, apricots, peppers, papaya, cantaloupe, tomatoes, broccoli, and blackberries. By the way, the key to getting bioflavonoids from citrus fruits is to eat the white part under the skin and around each segment of fruit. That is your richest source of bioflavonoids, so don't toss it away. Also, when you juice citrus fruits, don't throw away the pulp.

As a supplement, bioflavonoids are sold in combination with vitamin C. A vitamin C supplement made from rosehips contains naturally occurring bioflavonoids.

*How much should you take?*

While there is no established minimum daily requirement, nutritionists generally recommend between 200 to 900 mg on a daily basis.

### 91 Use vitamin A for *All* of you—from skin to within.

"A" stands for all-over health. Vitamin A is responsible for healthy skin, teeth, and hair. But its benefits are more than skin-deep. At the genetic level, vitamin A helps to build RNA, the very fabric of our makeup.

Vitamin A is perhaps best known for preventing night blindness. But it does so much more than that. Recently, vitamin A has been recognized as having potent anticancer properties. By keeping cell membranes strong, this antioxidant vitamin makes it more difficult for tumors to enter cells. So smokers, for instance, who take sufficient amounts of A lower their chances of getting lung cancer. (This is not to say you should feel free to smoke, or indulge in any other body-wrecking habit, and then dose yourself with vitamins to offset the bad effects! That approach to health does not work.)

Vitamin A also protects its users against the effects of physical and psychological stress. If you live in a polluted metropolitan area, it's wise to take extra A for protection against the heavy metals, carbon monoxide, ozone, and other harmful substances that you're inhaling daily. Combine the A with vitamins C and E and you will feel even better.

Moreover, vitamin A keeps you sexy. The health of your reproductive system, including your fertility and sperm production, depends on it.

### What happens if you don't get enough vitamin A?

Signs of a vitamin A deficiency include fingernails that break easily or grow slowly and that lack a pink tinge under the nail, frequent infections, night blindness, cloudy vision, itchy dry eyes and ulcers of the cornea (the transparent front part of the eye), dry skin, dry and brittle hair, and skin rashes. In children, slow growth and poor appetite may be signs of vitamin A deficiency.

### Where can you get vitamin A?

Animal products containing vitamin A are butter, milk, cheese, and egg yolk. Vegetable sources include yellow or orange fruits and vegetables such as sweet potatoes, carrots, turnips, apricots, and peaches. It's also found in spinach, beet and collard greens, kale, prunes, and tomatoes.

You've probably heard of beta carotene. It's a substance that the body can partially convert into vitamin A, and it's contained in vegetables. Beta carotene protects the immune system, especially the thyroid gland. To get more beta carotene, drink some carrot juice each day.

### How much vitamin A should you take?

The average person in good health should be getting 4,000 to 7,000 I.U. (international units) of vitamin A, or 5,000 to 10,000 I.U. of beta carotene daily. If you're already getting beta carotene from vegetables, you need less vitamin A than the amount suggested here. Vitamin A's benefits are enhanced by the addition of vitamin E and zinc.

Note: Since vitamin A is fat-soluble, it is stored by the body and not excreted through the urine or perspiration. Too much, therefore, can be toxic. Pregnant women, and those who may become pregnant, should be especially careful. Although vitamin A is an essential nutrient for babies' development, an excess of this vitamin taken early in pregnancy can cause birth defects. Of course, all pregnant women should see their health care practitioners for guidance on nutrition and other concerns, but the general recommendation on vitamin A is that those who are, or may become, pregnant should not take daily supplements containing more than 4,000 to 8,000 I.U. Beta carotene, though, found in vegetables, fruits, and some supplements, is not a problem. The body converts it to vitamin A at safe levels only.

### 92 Use E for energy.

If you want to remain young, healthy, and energetic, make sure to get enough vitamin E. This vitamin's other name, tocopherol, means ability to reproduce, which is an apt name for a nutrient that rejuvenates within and without.

Vitamin E, like a partner in marriage, is with you both in sickness and in health. If you suffer from a heart, respiratory, muscle, skin, or blood disease, vitamin E gets you on the road to health. It is also an important nutrient to take when fighting cancer. If you are healthy, it increases your sense of well-being and vitality. As an antioxidant, vitamin E keeps cells strong and disease-resistant. In today's world, our cells are constantly bombarded by contaminants, and vitamin E is great at guarding cells from their damaging effects. Since healthy cells are what keep you young, vitamin E, in effect, slows down the aging process.

*What if you don't get enough vitamin E?*

If you are deficient in vitamin E, you may get

edema (swelling) in the face, ankles, or legs; you may also experience poor skin condition, cold fingers and toes from poor circulation, muscle cramps, an abnormal heartbeat, or respiratory difficulties. And when blood tests reveal weakened, damaged red blood cells, lack of vitamin E may be the cause.

### Where can you get vitamin E?

Foods high in this supernutrient include wheat germ and wheat germ oil, polyunsaturated salad oils such as safflower and soy, unrefined whole grains, seeds, nuts, bran, and fertile organic eggs.

Concerning oils, you should know that heating, pasteurizing, filtering, and deodorizing oils are processes that remove most of the vitamin E. So use cold-pressed oils that have been minimally refined.

### How much should you take?

Due to the daily stresses of modern life, we can all benefit from a vitamin E supplement, especially since it protects against cancer. Besides, wouldn't you like to stay younger longer?

When searching for a supplement, choose one that reads "d-alpha-tocopherol." This tells you that it is natural and contains more active ingredients. The label "dl" means the vitamin was synthetically derived, and is thus less effective. Nutritionists and doctors recommend anywhere from 30 to 400 I.U. a day.

Note: If you have high blood pressure, see a physician before starting vitamin E.

## 93 Meet the vitamin B complex: It's a whole crew that helps you!

The B vitamins are a whole family of water-soluble nutrients that work as a team. The group includes $B_1$, $B_2$, $B_3$, $B_6$, $B_{12}$, biotin, pantothenic acid, choline, folic acid, inositol, and PABA.

The B complex crew works around the clock to

keep your body alive and well. They help enzymes release energy from foods and supplements, build healthy red blood cells, and keep cells supplied with oxygen. They detoxify the liver, protect against heart disease, and calm your nervous system. The B family also keeps your skin and hair healthy and promotes good vision.

As you can see, everyone needs the B complex vitamins, but they are especially important in higher amounts for alcoholics, pregnant women, and those with radiation sickness, constipation, intestinal discomfort, and cardiovascular disease. Orthomolecular physicians, doctors who specialize in vitamin therapy, have reported success when using megadoses of B vitamins in the treatment of schizophrenia and other mental illness.

### What happens if you don't get enough B vitamins?

If you aren't getting enough B vitamins you may have some of the following signs: skin rash, mouth sores, loss of appetite, poor muscle tone, chronic fatigue, depression, irritability and other nervous disorders, premature graying of the hair, and lowered resistance to colds and other infections.

Blood samples are the most accurate indicators of a B vitamin deficiency. Checking your tongue may also let you know: Usually, a pink tongue means that you are getting enough B vitamins, while a tongue that is dark or blue, with ridges, means you need higher amounts.

### What are good sources of B vitamins?

B vitamins are contained in brown rice and other whole grains; dried beans, especially soybeans; poultry; eggs; liver; fish; and fresh, leafy green vegetables, like spinach, turnip greens, broccoli, collards, dandelion, kale, mustard greens, cabbage, and cauliflower. Wheat germ, rice bran, and brewer's yeast are other rich vitamin B sources.

You should be aware that improper cooking can cause you to lose your B vitamins and other water-soluble nutrients. Instead of boiling fresh vegetables, try steaming them. If you do boil, though, use the cooking water in a sauce or soup and you'll still be a nutrient-wise chef.

### How much should you take?

While whole foods are your best B source, you can derive additional benefit from a supplement that contains the whole group of B vitamins in correct ratios. This is especially important if you are suffering from depression or another nervous system disorder, if you drink coffee or alcohol, or if you sweat a great deal. According to official sources, the average adult, between the ages of 23 and 50, should be getting these minimum daily requirements:

|  | *Males* | *Females* |
| --- | --- | --- |
| $B_1$ | 1.4 mg | 1.0 mg |
| $B_2$ | 1.6 mg | 1.2 mg |
| $B_3$ | 18.0 mg | 13.0 mg |
| Folic acid | 400.0 mcg | 400.0 mcg |
| $B_6$ | 2.0 mg | 2.0 mg |

## 94 Bone up on vitamin D.

Vitamin D is the "sunshine vitamin." We get it when sunlight enters the bloodstream through the pores of the skin. It is also a fat-soluble vitamin found in foods, and helps your body perform a variety of essential functions. It helps your body use calcium and phosphorus to form strong bones and teeth. It's also essential for healthy kidneys.

### What happens if you don't get enough vitamin D?

A lack of vitamin D causes bone diseases such as rickets (weak, deformed bones in the young) and osteoporosis (brittle, fragile bones in the old). It can also lead to kidney disease and failure.

### What are good sources?

One hour of direct sunlight each day will give you all the vitamin D you need. But since sun has gotten so much bad press these days from being linked to skin cancer, you may want to consider getting less sun and more vitamin-D-rich foods. Sources to consider include fish liver oils, butter, milk, egg yolk, sardines, salmon, tuna, and herring.

Children and older people, nursing mothers, and individuals living in a climate with little sunlight should consider taking a fish liver oil capsule as well.

### How much should you take?

Official sources recommend 400 I.U., or international units, daily. Greater amounts may be needed to build resistance against bone disease, and to treat patients suffering from rheumatoid arthritis, psoriasis, and tuberculosis, but megadoses of this supplement are not recommended. Vitamin D is a fat-soluble vitamin that is stored in the body, and too much can be toxic.

## 95 Learn about vitamin K—you may need more of it at some point.

Vitamin K is a little-known, fat-soluble nutrient that plays a vital role in the maintenance of healthy blood and bones. It is naturally produced by the intestines, but can be enhanced by the foods that we eat.

Vitamin K forms prothrombin, a protein made by the liver that helps blood to clot. This is important for your recovery from wounds. In addition, K helps keep bones strong.

### What happens if you don't get enough vitamin K?

Too little vitamin K is signified by a tendency to

bruise easily and an inability of the blood to coagulate. Premature infants who have not yet developed intestinal bacteria and whose mothers did not take an anticoagulant are at great risk for this problem.

### What are good sources?

Rich sources of vitamin K include green, leafy vegetables, such as kale and spinach. It is also found in cauliflower, broccoli, and cabbage. Foods that encourage healthy bacteria, such as yogurt, miso, and tempeh, help your body manufacture more of this vital nutrient.

Supplements are unavailable over-the-counter, but are sometimes prescribed for people who have blood clotting problems.

### How much should you take?

Little is known about how much vitamin K individuals need on a daily basis, but people who take chemical laxatives or have ulcerative colitis or diarrhea may need more than the average person does. It is also good to take extra K if you are about to undergo surgery. Its use in cancer is controversial, but it may be helpful. Whether or not it should be used, and exact amounts, should be determined by a nutritionally oriented physician.

## 96 Eat with calcium in mind.

Calcium is your chief mineral, constituting 2 percent of your body weight. Its main function is to build and maintain strong bones and teeth, but it has other valuable jobs as well. Did you know that every cell of yours bathes in calcium, because it's an important component of cell membranes? Additionally, calcium plays an active role in the production of hormones and in stimulating enzymes so that you can digest your food and contract your muscles. It's also needed for your circulatory and immune systems to function properly.

# VITAMINS, MINERALS, AND MORE

## What happens if you don't get enough calcium?

Symptoms of a calcium deficiency include nervousness, depression, headaches, and insomnia. A lack of calcium leads to problems with all major systems. The brain and muscles do not function properly, nor do the digestive, immune, and circulatory systems. Osteoporosis, the condition characterized by fragile bones, can be a problem in later life, particularly for women, if calcium is insufficient.

## What are good sources of calcium?

Calcium is found in milk and other dairy products such as buttermilk, yogurt, acidophilus milk, and cheese, and indeed, dairy products have traditionally been touted as the best calcium source. There are some problems, though, with relying on dairy for this purpose. One is that many people are allergic to dairy products. And, more fundamentally, although dairy foods *are* first in the quantity of calcium they contain, they aren't when you consider absorbability of the nutrient. When you consider that factor—how much of the food's calcium we can actually use—dark green vegetables, including sea vegetables, come out on top. Further, juicing your dark green vegetables—such as kale, parsley, collard greens, Swiss chard, and arugula—is even better than eating them in solid form when it comes to infusing your body with this vital nutrient. So you might want to consider replacing that glass of milk with a glass of mixed vegetable juice that's got some good green stuff in it.

Other calcium sources include oatmeal, tempeh, sesame seeds, and carob flour.

## How much should I take?

Healthy adults benefit from 800 mg daily. Pregnant and lactating women need 1,200 mg. Older women can benefit from calcium supplements in the form of amino acid chelate to prevent or fight osteoporosis.

## 97 Don't overlook magnesium.

Magnesium is a master mineral that ceaselessly works in your muscles, cells, nervous system, bones, digestive system, metabolism, reproductive system, protein production system, blood, and immune system. Whew! Did we get everything in? It's hard to, because magnesium is one of the body's most important co-enzymes whose main function involves making your metabolism as efficient as possible.

*What happens if you don't get enough magnesium?*

Signs of a magnesium deficiency include an irregular heartbeat, hair loss, nails that break easily, muscle cramping, and fatigue.

*What are good sources?*

The best foods for magnesium are leafy green vegetables such as kale, endive, chard, beet greens, alfalfa sprouts, and celery. Other rich sources include nuts and seeds, especially peanuts, pecans, almonds, cashews, Brazil nuts, hazelnuts, sunflower seeds, pumpkin seeds, and sesame seeds. A salad of leafy greens topped with nuts and slices of avocado is a great way to get your quota of magnesium for the day.

*How much should you take?*

It may be a good idea to take between 450 and 650 mg of magnesium for optimal health. Actually, it's a bit more complicated than that in that you should always consider magnesium in relation to calcium. Specifically, your calcium/magnesium ratio ought to be balanced at 1:1. Calcium citrate/magnesium citrate is a good source of both minerals in a balanced form. Take in between meals, as it might otherwise interfere with digestion.

## 98 Meet chromium: You need just a little of it, but you need it a lot.

Chromium? Isn't that the shiny trim on cars? Not exactly. It's a nutrient found in trace amounts in your body, and it's vital to your overall health.

Chromium supports the heart, liver, brain, and glucose metabolism. It helps insulin transfer glucose, or sugar, from the bloodstream to the cells, and it assists the liver in the removal of excess fats from the blood. It also aids in the production of protein and in the immune system's defense against toxins. Chromium counteracts stress and prevents premature aging. Plus it's been shown to aid in weight loss.

### What happens if you don't get enough chromium?

Signs of a chromium deficiency include fatigue, dizziness, anxiety, insomnia, a craving for alcohol, blurred vision, depression, and panic. Premature aging may occur as well.

### What are good sources of chromium?

You can get chromium from whole wheat flour, brewer's yeast, nuts, black pepper, whole grain cereals (except rye and corn), fresh fruit juice, dairy products, root vegetables, legumes, leafy vegetables, and mushrooms.

### How much should you take?

Nutritionists suggest taking a supplement of 200 mcg (micrograms) a day, especially if you have hypoglycemia, diabetes, heart disease, high cholesterol, poor eyesight, mental illness, or a susceptibility to infections. It's also important if you are exposed to heavy pollution, are recovering from surgery, are pregnant, or are suffering from arthritis. For weight loss, a chromium/niacin complex is sometimes used; it generally contains 200 mcg and 100 mg of those respective nutrients.

*SUPERCHARGE YOUR HEALTH!*

**99** **To keep your thyroid ticking, get enough iodine.**

Only a tiny fraction of our body weight is composed of iodine, but it helps us in many important ways. Most iodine is stored in the thyroid gland, where it creates thyroxin, a hormone mainly responsible for the speed at which we metabolize food. Thyroxin's other functions include the production of protein, the transformation of carotene into vitamin A, and protection from heart disease.

*What happens if I don't get enough iodine?*

Many people have underactive thyroids due to an iodine deficiency and don't even know it. The result? Sluggish behavior, forgetfulness, a lack of interest in sex, a poor complexion, and unhealthy teeth, hair, and nails. More severe indications are chronic fatigue, impotence, overweightness, irritability, and arthritis.

*What are good sources of iodine?*

If you want to prevent thyroid problems, try adding the iodine-rich sea vegetables to your diet. Use kelp in your homemade soups and dulse in your salads, or take kelp tablets for a more concentrated effect. Other food sources include iodized salt, fresh fish, garlic, dried mushrooms, and whole grain breads, muffins, and crackers. Some iodine is also present in leafy green vegetables, celery, tomatoes, radishes, carrots, bananas, strawberries, oranges, and grapefruits.

*How much should I take?*

If you choose to take an iodine supplement, 50 to 150 mcg is a safe amount. It is nontoxic, and what you don't use leaves the body.

**100** **Get enough iron—but not too much.**

You probably associate iron with rich blood, and rightly so. Iron makes hemoglobin, a compound that transports oxygen to your cells and turns blood bright red. It then acts as a garbage man by picking up carbon dioxide from your cells and carrying it back to your lungs so that you can breathe it out. In addition, iron allows muscle cells to produces energy. Finally, it helps an enzyme called ATP (adenosine triphosphate) to break down carbohydrates, fats, and proteins, and to store energy so that you don't use it up all at once.

### What happens if you don't get enough iron?

Signs of an iron deficiency may include chronic fatigue, shortness of breath, headaches, pale skin, and opaque or brittle nails.

### Where can you get it?

Nearly every food you eat contains iron. Especially good sources include egg yolks, leafy green vegetables, dried beans, peaches, apricots, dates, prunes, cherries, figs, raisins, and blackstrap molasses.

### When should you take supplemental iron?

If you are anemic, you may need additional iron. But you may not. For one thing, you may be anemic due to undetected internal blood loss; this should be investigated medically. Also, research reveals that there are several types of deficiency anemia besides that caused by lack of iron, like vitamin $B_{12}$, magnesium, copper, cobalt, or zinc deficiencies. Unfortunately, doctors sometimes prescribe iron for these other types of anemia, when too much can be dangerous, even fatal. Excess iron can cause heart problems, rheumatoid arthritis, cirrhosis, scurvy, low levels of vitamin E, respiratory and digestive problems, and even schizophrenia.

In addition to iron-deficiency anemia, instances in which extra iron may be needed are during pregnancy or after an accident in which blood was lost. Seek the guidance of a nutritionally knowledgeable health professional in supplementing iron.

*SUPERCHARGE YOUR HEALTH!*

## 101 Find out why selenium can help you function better and feel better.

Selenium, as an antioxidant, protects cells from destruction by oxygen. It's an anticancer mineral. It also helps the body's enzyme system and aids in protein production and in the manufacture of prostaglandins, which control blood pressure and clotting. Selenium also protects the eyes from cataracts and the arteries from plaque.

And if all that's not enough, consider that selenium can affect your mental outlook. A British study, reported on in the journal *Biological Psychiatry*, gave test subjects either selenium supplements or placebos, over a period of five weeks. Neither test subjects nor researchers knew who was getting what. The results showed that the selenium improved people's moods and decreased their anxiety levels. Plus those subjects who had lower initial levels of the nutrient were helped the most.

### What happens if you don't get enough selenium?

A selenium deficiency can occur from exposure to toxic chemicals, infections, digestive difficulties, allergies, and injuries. Also, different parts of the world have soils with varying selenium levels, which has repercussions as you go up the food chain. Signs of deficiency include wrinkles, sunken eyes, digestive problems, confusion, low blood pressure, irritability, difficult breathing, and heightened allergies. Subclinical levels of depression and anxiety resulting from less than optimum selenium intake might be hard to detect, but as we've just seen, there is a connection.

### What are good sources of selenium?

Eggs are excellent sources of selenium. So are other animal products. Plant sources include whole grains, mushrooms, asparagus, broccoli, onions, and tomatoes.

*How much should you take?*

Trace mineral experts recommend taking 75 to 150 mcg of chelated selenium daily. Selenium works well in combination with vitamin E.

### 102 Think zinc—for disease prevention and more.

Zinc may be last in the alphabet, but it shouldn't be last in your life. That's because this antioxidant trace mineral has so many important functions. It bolsters the immune system, and thus plays a role in fighting everything from cancer to colds. Zinc also plays an important role in the production of growth and sex hormones, and in the utilization of insulin. As a co-enzyme, zinc makes many vital contributions, including maintaining proper blood acidity, removing toxic metals, and helping the kidneys maintain proper mineral balance.

*What happens if you don't get enough zinc?*

Impaired ability to smell or taste is a sign of zinc deficiency, and, in fact, lack of this mineral is implicated as a factor in anorexia nervosa. Skin problems, such as stretch marks, acne, or psoriasis, are another sign.

*Where can you get zinc?*

Good zinc sources include eggs, poultry, and seafood, as well as peas, soybeans, mushrooms, whole grains, and nuts and seeds, especially pumpkin seeds.

*How much should you take?*

For adults, 20 to 25 mg daily is generally sufficient.

### 103 Remember manganese, please.

The nutrition world, like other aspects of our culture, has its media superstars—e.g., vitamin C, beta carotene, oat bran—that bask in the limelight and sometimes take on the aura of miraculous cure-alls that will solve our every health problem if we only take enough of them. Keep in mind, though, that magic bullets are rarely the solution to *any* health problem, and that we need a full spectrum of nutrients for our bodies to function optimally. Let's remember, for instance, the trace mineral manganese.

It hasn't made magazine covers, but the fact is that you need manganese for everything from your bones to your hormones. This mineral is essential to the production of protein and to the correct formation of your skeletal system, teeth, cartilage, and tendons. It transmits nerve impulses to your brain and creates new blood cells in the bone marrow. In addition, manganese is needed for the production of sex hormones, and the metabolism of blood sugar and fats.

### What happens if you don't get enough manganese?

Without manganese, blood sugar disorders and sexual dysfunction may develop. Low manganese is also connected to myasthenia gravis, a disease that deteriorates muscles, and to restricted protein production and carbohydrate/fat metabolism.

### What are good sources of manganese?

Good sources of manganese are nuts, seeds, whole grains, leafy green vegetables—particularly those that have been organically grown—rhubarb, broccoli, carrots, potatoes, peas, beans, pineapple, blueberries, raisins, cloves, and ginger.

### How much should you take?

Up to 7 mg daily of manganese is recommended as a supplement.

## 104 Understand sodium (salt)—but don't overdo it.

Sodium and potassium are partners that pump nutrients into cells, and get toxic waste out. Sodium also regulates fluid pressure in the cells, thus affecting blood pressure. Moreover, sodium helps control the acid/alkaline balance in the blood. It enables the nerves to transmit impulses to muscles that allow them to contract. It also helps to pump glucose into the bloodstream, produces hydrochloric acid for digestion, and keeps calcium suspended in the bloodstream, ready for use.

*What happens if you don't get enough sodium?*

Sodium deficiencies are rare, but may result from physical stresses, such as an exposure to toxic chemicals or injuries. Symptoms include wrinkles, sunken eyes, intestinal problems, confusion, fatigue, low blood pressure, irritability, breathing difficulties, and heightened allergies.

*Where can you get sodium?*

No need to seek this one out. Sodium is present in all the foods we eat, and in our water as well.

*How much do you need?*

You need between 55 and 440 mg of sodium each day, but—guess what!—you're probably getting a whole lot more. Most people consume between 7,000 and 20,000 mg daily, especially if they eat refined foods or add salt to their meals. Too much sodium can cause hypertension, or high blood pressure, stress, liver damage, muscle weakness, and pancreatic disease.

## 105 Remember potassium—particularly you runners.

Potassium works with sodium to form an electrical pump that speeds nutrients to all body cells and that carries out waste. It is also vital to the digestive and endocrine systems, as well as to the muscles, brain, and nerves. Potassium additionally helps to maintain the correct acid/alkaline balance of body fluids.

**SUPERCHARGE YOUR HEALTH!**

*What happens if you don't get enough potassium?*

Potassium deficiencies can result in slow healing, lethargy, insomnia, severe constipation, intestinal spasms, tissue swelling, thinning hair, and malfunctioning muscles. Most people get enough, but runners and other athletes who sweat a lot in training can get caught short on this one. Also, people taking diuretic medications may need extra.

*Where can you get potassium?*

The best sources are leafy green vegetables, bananas, cantaloupe, avocados, dates, prunes, dried apricots, raisins, whole grains, beans, legumes, and nuts and seeds. Meals based on grains and legumes can help athletes get what they need of this nutrient.

*How much should you take?*

Most diets don't supply all the potassium you need; if additional amounts are needed, consider adding 100–200 mg extra. A nutritionist can help determine if you need extra.

### 106 Hail phosphorus—for all of us!

All chances are you don't have to worry about this mineral because it's in so many foods. But that's one of the reasons you should be familiar with phosphorus; you've been seeing it on so many of the food labels you've been reading for nutritional information (you *have*, haven't you?). And you should appreciate phosphorus, too, because it plays such a big part in your body's functioning. Bones, teeth, nerves, muscles, the brain, liver, eyes, and the metabolic, cellular, digestive, and circulatory systems—all of these depend upon phosphorus. It's an essential part of your DNA and RNA and also helps to balance body fluids and to supply energy to muscles, which makes this mineral especially important for runners.

*What happens if you don't get enough phosphorus?*

Phosphorus deficiencies rarely occur, but when they do, they can cause a type of anemia and impair immunity.

*Where can you get it?*

This one's easy—practically everywhere. Sources include meat, poultry, fish, eggs, dairy products, whole grains, nuts and seeds, legumes, celery, cabbage, carrots, cauliflower, string beans, cucumber, chard, pumpkin, and fruits.

*How much do you need?*

Adults need 800 mg; pregnant and breast-feeding women need 1,200 mg. You're probably getting an adequate supply already.

## 107 Understand antioxidants.

We've mentioned antioxidants several times, and you've no doubt heard about them elsewhere. But what exactly are antioxidants, and why should we value them?

Antioxidants are compounds that work to neutralize free radicals. As to what *they* are, a free radical is a molecule that is missing an electron. Free radicals are highly reactive; they tend to steal electrons from normal molecules, which then themselves become free radicals in a chain reaction of oxidation. The result? Well, when all of this happens in your body you get various types of cellular damage, including lessened immune system function. Many age-associated bodily changes, including chronic diseases, are a result of free-radical-induced damage. By the way, free radicals are everywhere; you may have heard that they're generated by environmental pollutants, which is true, but they're also made by our own bodies.

It looks like a grim picture, but remember that

we have antioxidants, which will come in and quench free radicals, stopping the destructive reactions. That's why these substances are so valuable in the fight against premature aging and most of the illnesses we're faced with.

With all this in mind, let's briefly return to some of the nutrients we've looked at, to reinforce their status as antioxidants.

First, always remember these antioxidant vitamins—A, C, E; think of them as your disease-fighting ACE in the hole.

**VITAMIN A.** Did you know that vitamin A prevents the thymus gland from shrinking? This is important to immune defense, because the thymus manufactures T-cells, which are soldiers against tumors.

Related to vitamin A is its precursor, beta carotene (the substance that enables the body to produce the vitamin). Beta carotene stimulates interferon, T-helper cells, and natural killer cells, all vital elements in immune system defense. As an antioxidant, beta carotene may be more effective than vitamin A at protecting the thymus gland from free-radical damage.

**VITAMIN C.** Vitamin C aids in the manufacture of antibodies and white blood cells. It combats infections, viruses, and bacteria, helps the body to detoxify, and strengthens overall immune response.

Consider what an article in the *Journal of Advancement in Medicine* reported recently about the value of this vitamin as a sickness fighter. Groups of people were classified based on how much ascorbic acid (vitamin C) they consumed daily. Ingestion of less than 100 mg was associated with the greatest number of clinical signs and symptoms. Those who took 200 mg or more, by contrast, had the least symptomatology, in all age groups. And subjects over 50 who consumed the greatest amounts of vitamin C were clinically similar to 40-year-olds taking the least.

**VITAMIN E.** Vitamin E increases T-cells, B-cells, and natural killer cells. As an antioxidant, it prevents cellular damage caused by environmental poisons and other stressors, and is considered by nutritionally knowledgeable physicians to be vital in countering coronary heart disease.

Two other star antioxidants are in the mineral group.

**SELENIUM.** Clinical experience reveals time and again that people with low selenium levels are more likely to get cancer. This mineral raises immune status, detoxifies the system of poisons from the environment, protects the liver, and maintains cellular respiration.

Selenium works together with vitamin E.

**ZINC.** T-cells, antibodies, and natural killer cells need zinc, which are three reasons you shouldn't forget this antioxidant.

## 108 Meet glutathione peroxidase, superoxide dismutase, and catalase—and find out why they're your friends.

*What?!* I can hear you saying. *Maybe they're your friends, buddy, but they don't sound like mine. I don't even know what you're talking about.*

Okay, I'll start from the beginning. Glutathione peroxidase, superoxide dismutase, and catalase are three antioxidant enzymes. What's an enzyme? An enzyme is a catalyst; that is, it facilitates specific chemical reactions. The vitamins and minerals in our bodies need to link up with enzymes to do their work. Some enzymes, in addition to their function as catalysts, are free-radical scavengers, or antioxidants, as well.

**SUPERCHARGE YOUR HEALTH!**

Three enzymes have been noted to have remarkable antioxidant properties. They're glutathione peroxidase, superoxide dismutase (SOD), and catalase. All three are manufactured inside the body, and their job is to deactivate free radicals as they are formed. In doing so, they help to prevent numerous degenerative disorders, including heart disease, arthritis, neurological damage, and cancer. This also helps to keep us young.

Although enzymes are found naturally in our bodies, you can up your enzyme levels by eating live foods like sprouts, especially sunflower seed, lentil, mung bean, clover, radish, and mustard seed sprouts. It is also important to eat sulfur-containing foods, such as onions, eggs, and garlic, because glutathione needs sulfur amino acids to function as an antioxidant.

## 109 Look into the latest in nature's age-fighters.

They're not quite the answer to Ponce de Leon's dream, but they certainly would have caught his attention. I'm talking about the natural substances that, along with the more familiar vitamins and minerals, are being used today to combat age-related physical and mental changes. Unlike drugs, natural substances do not work instantaneously, so these compounds take awhile for their effects to be felt. But they have no side effects either, a very important plus. Here's a rundown on some substances that may slow your body's running down!

**ACETYL-L-CARNITINE.** This endogenous substance (meaning it's found naturally in the body) has been demonstrated to reverse age-related changes in the brain, which is why, today, many people are taking it to slow cerebral aging. They're not just acting on wishful thinking, because a mountain of research has come out that documents the power of carnitine to improve people's brain functioning. For instance, in one recent scientific study, elderly patients with failing motor and mental skills took the substance over a half-year period, with results of statistically significant upward trends in all performance areas, as well as an improved quality of life. In fact, researchers writing in the journal *Biological Psychiatry* feel that carnitine may be an effective long-term preventative agent to ward off mental deterioration.

**PHOSPHATIDYLSERINE.** Another substance that slows brain drain, phosphatidylserine has been shown in placebo-controlled studies to aid task performance and learning in elderly patients. Studies with rats document the actual brain-restorative action of this compound.

**GINKGO BILOBA.** Extracts of this herb have helped elderly subjects stem mental deterioration and thus stay out of nursing homes. In one double-blind, placebo-controlled trial, three months of taking ginkgo biloba yielded definite improvement in brain functioning. This safe and well-tolerated substance, researchers say, appears to fulfill the World Health Organization's criteria for a drug showing effectiveness against cerebral aging.

**MELATONIN.** This one's received a lot of publicity lately, but the media don't always stress that this is not a drug. Melatonin is a hormone that our brain's pineal gland produces normally. Levels fall with age, which can be a problem because this hormone helps in the regulation of sleep. Taking melatonin, though, has been shown to improve sleep quality, which, in turn, improves the quality of people's awake time. Another benefit of this substance: It's an antioxidant, so it works to scavenge free radicals and thus combat age-related degeneration.

**DHEA.** This hormone is found in higher levels in the young than in the old, and it's higher in the healthy than in the unhealthy. So it's been linked to our internal biological clock that determines life-span. Can extra DHEA keep that clock ticking longer? As of now, researchers do see potential in DHEA for combating cancer, lupus, AIDS, and other serious conditions. An important recent finding—demonstrated in a rigorously controlled study—is that DHEA improves feelings of well-being. People aged 40 to 70 were given DHEA supplements or a placebo. After two weeks, those receiving the DHEA felt significantly better than control-group members, both physically and psychologically.

**COENZYME Q–10.** Q–10 has proven of value in treating heart conditions and may help us maximize our lifespan, and energize it as well. "Senior citizen" mice fed the compound tend to live longer than their non-Q-10-fed peers, and they're more active in their old age as well. As an antioxidant, Q-10 works to detoxify LDL cholesterol (the bad kind), and it enhances the efficacy of vitamin E.

**QUERCETIN.** This is a bioflavonoid, one with real disease-fighting power. It knocks out cancer-causing agents, protects the DNA of our cells, and blocks enzymes that promote the growth of tumors. Quercetin is also effective against bacteria and viruses, as well as allergies.

## 110 Remember. . . *real* food first.

Once you've learned about the important nutrients, there may be the temptation to take a nutritional shortcut by cutting down on real food while taking a bunch of vitamin and mineral supplements.

Don't. While some supplement powders contain most of what you need for nourishment and can at times be used in place of food, vitamin and mineral pills can't. They are intended as add-ons to your meals, not as substitutes for them.

There are so many reasons you need real food, particularly plant-derived food. One is, of course, that you need the energy in it—the calories. (Well, you do need *some*!) Another is that you need the protein. Another is that you need the fiber in plant food, for digestive health. Yet another is that you need the phytochemicals in food, those hundreds of disease-fighting chemicals found in plants that can't possibly be replicated in supplements. Then too, you can't create a pleasant, sense-satisfying experience with a pill bottle the way you can with, say, a pasta and broccoli dish seasoned with garlic, flanked by a crisp green salad, and accompanied by warm whole-grain bread.

Yes, we've seen that there are problems with a lot of the food sold in supermarkets today. You can partially counter that by buying organically grown food, when possible. By definition, no pesticides or artificial fertilizers are used in the growth of organic produce. In the case of organically produced animal products, the animals used are fed organically grown grain, without additives, and they aren't given growth hormones. Plus organic farmers are more likely than others to care about the quality of their soil, which is important not just in terms of the vegetables we're eating today, but in terms of those that will be available for our children years down the road. Finally, but not least importantly, animals on organic farms are more likely to be treated in a humane way, e.g., to be given more space, freedom of movement, and sunshine than others.

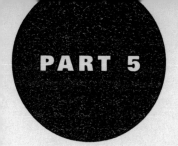

# PART 5

# THE HOWS AND WHYS OF EXERCISE

*Eating wholesome foods is a start. Taking the right supplementary nutrients is a help. But to really supercharge your health, exercise is essential. Here's all you need to know to get moving, and to keep motivated, too.*

## 111 Give yourself—and those who love you—the gift of exercise.

If you are like most Americans, you don't feel there are enough hours in the day to fit in a "frill" like exercise. Perhaps you have a family to care for, a full-time job, and other responsibilities. And even if you had the time, where would you get the energy?

Well, there's a happy paradox that you should be aware of: Exercise *makes* energy! The fact is making time for exercise gives you an extra boost. If you work out first thing in the morning or after work, you won't feel like hitting the couch when you get home. Instead, you will feel energized. So you'll have gained time. This is time you can use to read, study, work, or be with friends and family.

How exactly does expending energy increase energy? The explanation is simple. An aerobic workout sends additional oxygen to your brain, which keeps you feeling more alert.

Exercise also puts you in a better mood, because it helps prevent wide swings in blood sugar. If you feel selfish about taking time out for yourself, just consider that your improved frame of mind is a gift to the people you live with. Live alone? You still need to be good to yourself.

Another gift that you can give to yourself, and to the people who care about you, is better health and a longer life. This is one of the reasons I don't consider exercise a frill at all, but a basic necessity. Recent studies indicate that a quarter of a million Americans die each year indirectly from a lack of physical activity. Working out can prevent you from becoming a part of these statistics. Conversely, not working out increases your chances of a shortened or sickness-plagued life. I would even go so far as to say that not working out means that your *life's* not working out, at least not as well as it could.

Look at it from a negative standpoint for a moment. If you don't work out, you're going to have a weak and flabby body. What does this mean? First, you feel blah. Second, being weak and flabby opens you up to health problems. Plus remember that the flabbier you are, the more difficult it becomes to improve your health by losing weight. When you have too much fat on reserve, and do not exercise on a regular basis, your muscles begin to deteriorate, and fat infiltrates the tissues. The fat inside the muscles is known as intramuscular fat. As fat takes the place of muscles, you lose strength and stamina, and become increasingly prone to diseases and injuries. Plus, as fat accumulates, your life tends to become increasingly sedentary, in a vicious cycle that ends up with your doing less and less just when you should be doing more.

It may come as a surprise to learn that the extra weight that shows up on the scales is an advanced stage of a problem that has been with you for at least two years. The intramuscular fat, described above, settles first. The bulges on your buttocks, hips, thighs, and underarms show up later. If you try to get rid of them through dieting alone, you will never succeed, since fat-filled muscles cannot burn calories efficiently. The bottom line: You've got to incorporate exercise into your life, and the sooner, the better.

## 112 Get motivated to get moving.

Consider this: Once you're in shape you are able to engage in more physically challenging activities that make life fun. Also, once you feel and look better, you are increasingly eager to get out and enjoy the company of others.

This became apparent to me recently, after I

asked a group of friends to join me on a bike trip in New England. We would be going first through Martha's Vineyard and Cape Cod, and then alongside Maine's beautiful shoreline. Everybody thought this was a great idea, but out of the 15 people I originally asked to come along, only two ended up joining me.

Beyond all the excuses, I realized the genuine reason. Most of my friends didn't feel fit enough to go on this trip. Here were 13 people who would have loved doing something different and enjoyable, but who felt physically limited.

I suggested that they start to get in shape so that we could try this again in three months, and that motivated some people. About six of my friends realized that they were missing out on a chance to share camaraderie and to see new places. They started an exercise program to get themselves into condition.

Think of all the activities that you haven't done because you were out of shape. I'm not just talking about things like long-distance bike trips and mountain-climbing adventures, but even simple outings like going to the beach with friends, or taking a wilderness walk. Think of the dances you haven't gone to where you could have socialized. Think of the people you haven't allowed yourself to meet. Think of the clothes you could be wearing.

And as you project into the future, you might want to consider that a broad spectrum of ailments associated with aging can be reversed with exercise. By strengthening bones and muscles, osteoporosis (calcium loss from bones) may be prevented. This is great news for women, who from the age of 35 until menopause can lose up to 2 percent of the calcium in their bones yearly, and after menopause, as much as 5 percent each year.

### SUPERCHARGE YOUR HEALTH!

Working out is great for your heart, and as your cardiovascular system improves so does the rest of your body. Here's how all the improvement happens: Exercise results in the enlargement of blood vessels and arteries, which means that more blood flows to your organs and tissues; this prevents cells from dying and prolongs life. More oxygen gets to the brain, so your mind is clear, instead of confused and senile. At the other end of the body, wavelike movements in the intestine, called peristalsis, speed up. You are less constipated; therefore, byproducts of food exit your body quickly, and you are less prone to diseases like colorectal cancer, diverticulitis, and spastic colon. These are just a few of the reasons why if you keep moving, you slow down aging, and enjoy life more in the process as well.

### 113 Feel down? Rev up!

Exercise increases blood circulation to the brain, and lowers blood pressure. It also reduces muscle tension and prevents problems that a tense body can create. Studies show that psychological problems are handled better by the physically fit, and that they tend to suffer less from depression.

If depression already exists, exercise can have a great impact in overcoming it. No, exercise is not a cure-all, and people who are suffering from clinical depression should be under a doctor's care. But doctors do report that if depressed patients can get moving physically, the depression is usually alleviated somewhat. The problem is of course that activity is generally the last thing a depressed person feels like doing. But if he or she can somehow ease into an exercise program, however modest, the rewards will be more energy, a clearer mind, and very possibly a renewed interest in life.

## 114 Look at your exercise history—*is* there one?

Exercise should be a routine part of your life, like brushing your teeth. If it's not, explore the reasons why. There are many reasons you may have chosen not to exercise. Perhaps you felt fatigued or depressed, or were just not in the habit of working out. Perhaps you bought into old assumptions about exercise, such as that only the overweight need it. Just as you examined your upbringing to see how your eating patterns developed, look back to see how your attitude toward exercise came about.

If you've basically been a nonexerciser up till now, ask yourself why. Was there too much competition attached to exercise when you were growing up? Was it presented in gym class as something uncomfortable, or boring? Was it something that girls didn't have to be concerned with? Or that people who worked with their heads, and not their hands, didn't spend time on? We know all these attitudes are outdated, but perhaps their vestiges are still with you.

If you have been a nonexerciser, it's best to start slowly; you can begin by simply walking. In a short time, you will look forward to working out, and before you know it you will miss the days you skip.

## 115 Understand the different types of exercise.

We've all heard of aerobic exercise, and with good reason, because this is the type of conditioning that's vital for everyone. Aerobics is defined as any physical exercise that makes the heart and lungs work harder to meet the muscles' need for oxygen. Increased levels of oxygen improve the heart and lungs, and overall body functioning is ultimately improved. So is endurance.

## *SUPERCHARGE YOUR HEALTH!*

Running, walking, swimming, bicycling, and cross-country skiing are some of the exercises that fall into the aerobics category. These activities can be quite strenuous, but if you gradually build up, you will improve your body's ability to handle the stress. And that's a major part of what fitness is all about.

Another type of exercise is anaerobics. Anaerobic exercises will not replace the conditioning supplied by aerobics, but they are good at building strong, well-toned muscles. Anaerobics differ from aerobics because they do not require extra oxygen; they rely on energy stored in the muscles. The exercise usually has a duration of three to four minutes. Sprinting, golf, weight lifting, and wrestling are classic examples of anaerobic activity. To improve specific muscle groups, you can either choose two types of aerobic exercise or use one aerobic and one anaerobic activity. Some sports qualify as both. If you move continuously while playing tennis, for example, the exercise is aerobic. The quick, intense motion it takes to serve the ball is anaerobic.

Moving on in the quest for bodily perfection, are you familiar with isometrics, isotonics, and isokinetics? These three are muscle-toning exercises; that is, they increase the size and strength of particular muscles.

To perform isometrics, you raise muscle tension by putting pressure against stable resistance. This may be done by opposing different muscles in your own body, such as when you press your hands together, or by pushing or pulling against an immovable object. These exercises involve no joint movement.

In isotonics, you partially contract one muscle and then hold it in position, as in weight training. Unlike isometrics, isotonics do involve the movement of joints.

With isokinetics you apply constant force during motion. An example would be using the Nautilus machine; here you lift and lower weights with your own muscle power, rather than let gravity take the weight down, as happens with isotonic exercises. When the muscle reaches a partial resting position, the machine adds some resistance to force the muscle to exert energy.

### 116 Push those poisons out with aerobic exercise!

We've talked about detoxification from a nutritional standpoint. But did you know that an uninterrupted half hour of aerobic exercise, performed on a routine basis, is an excellent aid to detoxification? That's why, whenever you're detoxing, aerobics should be part of your program.

Again, aerobic exercise is the kind that makes the heart and lungs work harder to meet the muscles' need for oxygen. Thus, it results in improved heart and lung functioning. But at the same time, it works as an internal cleansing mechanism.

Activities such as walking, biking, swimming, and rowing rake up the residuals of detoxification and push them out of the body. Exercise also increases the efficiency of the lymphatic system, a network that extends throughout the entire body and that, as one of its functions, removes debris from the tissues.

### 117 Get medical clearance before embarking on an exercise program.

Don't suddenly start demanding a lot from your body without knowing what it is capable of doing. If you have a heart condition or are over 35, it is especially important to get a physical examination before you begin. Even if you are not in this category, tests can help you improve your nutritional status and prevent problems from showing up later on.

Your pre-exercise assessment should include a variety of tests, some of which we've mentioned in the previous section. Here are a few ways that a doctor can evaluate you with an eye to your exercise routine:

**PATIENT HISTORY.** Information obtained here includes personal and family medical history, allergies to foods and chemical substances, and other relevant factors such as smoking, medications, and psychological stress.

**PHYSICAL EXAMINATION.** This is an inspection for obvious medical concerns. A physical exam determines your current level of functioning and can uncover undetected illnesses. Your height and weight, blood pressure, and pulse are all important information here.

**BLOOD CHEMISTRY.** These tests measure blood sugar levels, thyroid function, cholesterol, including HDL and LDL, triglycerides, and protein, as well as digestive and absorptive capacity, liver and kidney function, and cardiac risk. They can reveal asymptomatic diseases, and are especially important if you have heart disease or a circulatory disorder.

**VITAMIN AND MINERAL ASSAYS (NUTRISCAN).** This test measures nutrient levels in the body and lets you know exactly what your body needs. Recent research shows that a lack of various nutrients can put you at risk for several disorders, including heart disease and cancer. Everyone can benefit from this test.

**URINALYSIS.** This test evaluates the amount of protein, sugar, bacteria, and ketones in the urine, and provides indirect information on kidney function, diabetes, and urinary tract infections. This is important because exercise stresses the kidneys.

**ELECTROCARDIOGRAM.** An electrocardiogram, or EKG, evaluates the electrical function of the heart, specifically the rate and rhythm of the heartbeat. If you have irregular beats when you rest or exercise, this may be a factor in how much strenuous activity you can engage in.

**HALTER MONITOR.** This test gives even more detailed information about heartbeat.

**STRESS TEST.** In this test, you walk on a treadmill while an EKG measures your heartbeat. If you are about to engage in strenuous physical activity, you should consider this test, especially if you are over 35.

**DOPPLER SONOGRAPHY.** Sound waves produce a picture of the organs and vessels, thereby revealing any abnormal masses, tumors, or deposits of plaque on the blood-vessel walls.

**118** **Determine your target heart rate range; then work out within it for 20 to 30 minutes, at least three days a week.**

For any aerobic exercise program, you need to determine your target heart rate so that you know how far to push yourself. What this refers to is the number of times you want your heart to beat per minute, as you exercise. Target heart rate is a range, not one number.

Your optimal range is simple to calculate. First, obtain your maximum heart rate by subtracting your age from 220. (Your *real* age, please—you don't have to let anybody else see this!) Then figure out 60 percent and 80 percent of your maximum rate. When you exercise aerobically, you need to stay within this target range.

**SUPERCHARGE YOUR HEALTH!**

## HOW TO DETERMINE YOUR HEART RATE
## (FOR 40-YEAR-OLD)

Maximum Rate
$220 - 40 = 180$

Low Target
$180 \times 0.60 = 108$

High Target
$180 \times 0.80 = 144$

While exercising, check your wrist for a pulse count to make sure that you are between your low and high target rates. If your pulse is too low, get it up a bit; if it is too high, slack up.

You will only benefit from your program if you stay within this range. When you exceed the 80-percent mark, you are placing too much stress on your system, and can even cause a heart attack. If you are working below your target rate, you are not exercising hard enough to profit aerobically from the activity.

When you exercise, begin gradually, and build up to your target rate. (Warm-up exercises, which we'll discuss next, will help prepare you for a workout.) The most aerobic gain occurs within the first 20 or 30 minutes of exercise. So your best plan is to exercise at your target heart rate for 20 to 30 minutes, three or more days a week.

Monitoring how you're doing is easy, and will give you a sense of accomplishment. At the beginning, to get an accurate measure of your heart rate you'll want to check your pulse for a full 60 seconds. But then, as you get into the swing of exercising and periodically monitoring your heart rate, instead of measuring your pulse for a full minute you can do so for 15 seconds and then multiply by

4. After awhile you'll gain an internal feel for when you're within the correct range. Do monitor regularly, though, just to be sure.

## 119 Always warm up before you start your aerobic activity.

You know that great motivational saying, "Just do it"? Well, with aerobics, we've got to modify that to "Just do it—but first, warm up," and also, "Just do it—but then, cool down." The fact is that just jumping into an aerobic activity is foolish. If you want to enhance your performance, and prevent muscle stress and strain that leads to injury, you need to warm up before aerobic exercise and cool down afterwards. Warm-up and cool-down exercises are easy to do, and they can in fact become a relaxing, enjoyable part of your routine. A total program that gives you a comprehensive workout will enhance your entire well-being, so always think in terms of easing into, and out of, your aerobic activity.

Let's look at warm-ups. Some novice exercisers think of these gentle movements as a frill that can be dispensed with. But the value of a pre-exercise routine cannot be overstated. Muscle injuries commonly result from poor circulation and cold muscles, both of which can be avoided through proper warm-up. Studies demonstrate a link between warming up and not hurting yourself during exercise.

As you warm up, a number of good things happen. More blood reaches your muscles, tendons, and ligaments, making them pliable, and better able to withstand pressure. In addition, the strength and speed of your muscles improve, allowing them to perform their full range of motion. You also save energy, and since you use less energy to work out, you can exercise longer. Moreover, nutrients reach muscles quicker, and exercise-induced lactic acid, which can cause cramping, leaves the body more easily.

When you prepare for your workout, you lessen your chance of getting a heart attack. If you exercise too strenuously, too soon, without warming up, you can place too much stress on your heart— even if you are in good condition. Research reveals that 75 percent of people who exercise without such precautions show abnormal tracings on electrocardiograph tests.

## 120 Start your warm-ups with deep breathing.

Your warm-ups should ideally consist of four light activities: (1) deep breathing; (2) warming up major muscle groups; (3) loosening your joints; and (4) stretching. Let's start with step 1, deep breathing:

Stand, lie on your back, or sit comfortably. Your head, neck, and spine should be in a straight line. Rest your hands on your lower abdomen and gently close your eyes. As you inhale slowly and deeply, your diaphragm pushes against your hands as it expands; as you exhale, its size decreases. Repeat 5 to 10 times. After you are completely relaxed, slowly open your eyes. Then take your pulse to get your resting heart rate. (You'll be referring to this after cool-down, to get your recovery time.)

A few tips about optimal warm-up breathing:
• Inhaling and exhaling should be done through the mouth.
• Do not move your chest and shoulders as you breathe.
• To release tensions in specific muscles, visualize

the breath going to those areas. With each exhalation, imagine the tension leaving that part of your body.

• While you are still relaxed, it's a good time to visualize yourself successfully performing your activity. Studies show that athletes who imagine success perform consistently better than those who do not.

### 121 By the way, learn how to breathe.

How to breathe?! Doesn't everyone know how? Maybe, but if you are like the average person, you could benefit from a few breathing lessons and improve your everyday technique. Most people take several shallow breaths per minute. The right way to breathe is slowly, and from the abdomen.

Try this. Inhale slowly as you expand your abdomen slightly. As you exhale, it will be somewhat depressed. At first, this may feel forced, but in a short while, you will feel natural with the method.

The advantages? Breathing deeply and fully creates a maximum exchange of oxygen and carbon dioxide. As a result you have more energy, and less fatigue.

Keep in mind that breathing exercises also help the nervous system, and they're an essential part of yoga practice. If you need to improve focus, concentration, and mental clarity, try yoga.

### 122 Warm up major muscle groups (step 2 of your warm-ups).

For the second phase of your warm-ups, spend a couple of minutes going nowhere. What I mean is, walk in place or lie on your back and bicycle in place with your legs in the air for 2 to 5 minutes.

Additionally, if you have no problems with your

heart, you can do gentle sit-ups as well to strengthen your abdominals and help improve posture. But they must be done the right way.

### 123 Loosen your joints, from head to toe (step 3 of your warm-ups).

These exercises activate synovial fluid, which lubricates joints and ligaments, thereby protecting them from getting strained as you exercise. If you have joint problems, doing these exercises in a pool will allow you freer range of motion. Perform these exercises slowly, never forcing them.

Note: If you can't visualize a new exercise, you need to read instructions to do it the first few times. Don't let that put you off, or give you the idea that these warm-up moves are complicated. They're not. Movements here should be relaxed, and require very little effort.

**SHOULDERS.** Raise your shoulders and let them fall 10 times, in a shrugging motion. Move your shoulders back and forth 10 times as well. Place one arm straight out in front of you. Turn it gently, in a complete circle, 10 times in one direction, and 10 times in the other. Repeat with the other arm. Place both arms out to the side and repeat the exercise, only this time turn both arms in the same direction at the same time.

**ELBOWS.** With arms outstretched in front of you, palms up (as if you are holding onto dumbbells), curl your arms toward your body, at the same time. Then lower them gently. Repeat 10 times. Repeat this exercise with the palms facing downward.

**WRISTS.** Clasp the hands and bend them from left to right, as you gently bend the wrists back and forth. Repeat 10 times in each direction. Next, grasp your left wrist with your right hand, and rotate the left hand in a circle. Relax the wrist that's being held, and pretend to draw a circle with your index finger. Complete the circle 10 times clockwise and 10 times counterclockwise. Repeat the exercise with the other wrist.

**FINGERS.** Make a soft, relaxed fist with each hand by gently folding your fingers in your palm. Open and close both hands in a gentle fist 10 times.

**HIPS.** Stand with feet shoulder-width apart. Rotate your hips in a slow, gentle circle, as if you are using a hula hoop, 10 times in each direction.

**KNEES.** Ankles, knees, and feet are touching as you bend slightly forward at the knees. Do not bend very deeply. Place your hands on top of your kneecaps and rotate them in a slow circle. Move your buttocks and knees together. Do this 10 times clockwise and 10 times counterclockwise. Pretend that a pen extends straight out from your kneecaps, and that you are trying to draw a circle with it.

**ANKLES.** Sit on a chair or on the floor, and place your left ankle on top of your right thigh, close to the knee. Hold your left leg just above the ankle with your left hand, and use your right hand to grasp your left foot by the toes, and rotate the foot. Your ankle should be loose as your hand does the work. Never rotate your ankle by using your leg muscles. Repeat 10 times in each direction, and repeat with the other ankle.

**METATARSALS.** Use your right hand to grasp the ball of your left foot. Flex the metatarsal joints (which stretch from the toes to the top of the foot) straight up and down 10 times, mimicking the motion of walking. Then do the same for each toe individually. Switch and repeat with the right foot and toes. In addition, spend a few minutes massaging the top and bottom of each foot. The massage will stimulate the circulation to your feet. Using your fingers and palms, knead your feet in a circular motion, applying gentle pressure.

## 124 Stretch (step 4—the last—of your warm-ups).

Now that you've warmed up a bit and loosened your joints, you are ready for a few muscle stretches. Always stretch after your other warm-ups to avoid injury to cold muscles. The focus is on passive stretching—relaxed, gentle muscle extensions that enhance flexibility—not bouncing motions that tighten, and may tear, muscles.

In the following exercises, stretch continuously and hold the end position from 10 to 30 seconds. Use your hands and arms, rather than your body weight, to control the stretch. Stay relaxed. To obtain more of a stretch, gently bend into the stretch as you exhale, but never force yourself to do more than you can do.

**QUADRICEPS.** This exercise stretches the muscles in front of the thighs. Placing your right hand against a wall, hold the top of your left foot with your left hand. Now pull your foot straight up behind you until it touches your buttock. Be sure that your leg is not twisted to the side, and that the left thigh is in front of the right thigh, not even with it. Hold for 20 seconds as you gently pull it up. Repeat 2 to 5 times for each leg. This leg stretch can also be performed while lying on your side.

**BUTTOCKS AND HAMSTRINGS.** This exercise helps alleviate stress on the lower back and stretches upper rear leg muscles. Lie on the floor and bend your right knee. Place both hands behind the knee (never on top of the knee or it may slip). Pull your knee toward your chest and lift your head slightly, as if you were going to kiss the knee. Hold that position for 20 seconds. Lower foot and leg completely to the floor. Then repeat the stretch 5 times for each leg. Slow down if you feel any strain on your legs or back. This exercise should not cause you any pain.

**LOWER LEGS AND FEET.** This towel stretch helps the lower rear leg and foot muscles. Sit on the floor with your legs extended straight out in front of you and your feet pointing up. Sling a towel or belt around the bottom of your right foot, as you hold the ends in your hands. Slowly lean backwards toward the floor, keeping your legs relaxed, your heels on the floor, and your back straight.

As you perform this exercise, your leg will move toward your face. Your upper body should be performing the work, and your legs should be very relaxed. If you feel any discomfort, be more relaxed. Hold for 20 seconds. Repeat 3 to 5 times for each leg.

Now you are ready to walk, run, jump, swim, ski, bike, or row.

### 125  Improve your sit-up smarts.

Many people do sit-ups incorrectly. As a result, they get no benefit from the exercise, and may even cause lower-back damage. Here are a few types of sit-ups you can do, and the proper way to do them.

• *Start with the stomach crunch; it's the gentlest form of sit-up:* Lie on your back, feet on the floor. Knees are bent and touching one another. Rest your hands on your shoulders or across the chest, but do not place them behind your head or neck. Lift your head and raise your shoulder blades just a few inches off the floor, only enough to feel it in your stomach. Repeat this several times.

• *As you get stronger, you can progress to the next level with this style of sit-up:* Exhale as you sit up a few inches. Do not lift your shoulders more than 10 inches. Hold for 10 seconds and then lower shoulders back to the floor. Repeat 5 to 10 times. If you have no problem with this exercise, try the normal bend sit-up.

• *Normal bend sit-ups are done quickly.* Exhale as you raise your head and shoulders, inhale as you lower them. Keep your head off the ground until you are finished. Keep your movements rhythmic to warm up the abdominal muscles. Start slow with 10 to 20 repeats. In the second week, add more.

## 126 Choose an aerobic activity that you enjoy.

In gym class, you probably had no choice. But in life, you do. So choose an exercise that you like and you will feel more motivated to stay with it. Better yet, choose two. Doing the same exercise all the time can become tedious. It's nice to have a change of pace. Also, combining different exercises uses more muscles throughout the body. Since aerobic conditioning is your primary goal, alternate between two types of aerobic exercises, or choose one aerobic activity and one anaerobic.

Remember that how much you benefit from an aerobics program depends upon how long, how often, and how hard you work. How long you exercise depends on your present conditioning and progress, and how often depends, of course, on your schedule, with three to five days a week being your parameters. As for intensity, you will need to measure your heart rate and stay within your target range. As we've mentioned, working out within your target heart rate range three to five days a week, for 20 to 30 minutes each time, is your goal.

Don't forget to perform pre- and post-exercise routines to enhance the activity itself, and to decrease the chance of injury.

### 127 Exercise isn't just jumping-jacks anymore: Consider your aerobic alternatives.

Did you ever hear someone say they hate to exercise? Maybe you've even said it yourself. When I hear this, I have to conclude that the person just hasn't found the right exercise yet, because there are so many types to choose from that it would be impossible not to find *something* to like. People may be stuck in the mindset of the past, when exercise was just about synonymous with calisthenics, but today, our concept of exercise has broadened so much that there's something for virtually everyone to enjoy.

Read through the next few pages to see what exercise options sound enjoyable to you. And as you read, keep in mind that you have choices not only about the exercise forms you engage in, but also about the conditions under which you engage in them: You can exercise in peaceful solitude or while enjoying the company of others; you can find excitement in friendly rivalry, or compete only with yourself. You can even forget about competition altogether and just go with the flow. When you tailor a program that's perfectly suited to your tastes, personality, and energy level, you'll get fit sooner and keep fit longer. So it's worth really thinking through your exercise options.

### 128 Get on the fast track to health— run!

A few decades ago, any adult seen running through an American neighborhood who wasn't trying to catch a train or escape from danger would have been considered a nut. Today, people bent on improving their health—and their state of mind— are seen running through the streets all the time.

Even Presidents do it! Our national acceptance, and even embracing, of this activity is truly one of the ways our world has improved over the past 20 or 30 years.

Running is a popular sport for several reasons. It is easy to do, and produces results quickly. Thirty minutes of running offers the same heart benefits as 90 minutes of walking. Moreover, the activity can be performed year-round, out of doors, or indoors on a treadmill. What's more, except for a good pair of running shoes, your investment in equipment is inexpensive. Makes you want to get out there and jog, doesn't it? Before you put on your running shoes and take off, there are a few things you should know:

- *Start slowly and gradually build up speed*. Running too fast too soon can place undue stress on the heart.
- *Be conscious of your running form*. Your back should be straight, with your body bent forward just slightly, and your head should be level; you shouldn't be looking down at your feet. "Look down, slow down; look up, speed up," is a jingle that helps beginning runners to focus outward. Bend your arms slightly and allow them to swing gently at the waist in a forward/backward motion. Your hands should be relaxed, with your fingers gently closed. To soften and distribute your body's impact, be sure to hit the ground with the heel and then roll the foot from heel to toe.
- *Invest in good running shoes*. Choose a quality pair that protect your feet and body. You do not need the most expensive brand; a good shoe priced in the middle range will do. And remember that every so often you will need to invest in a new pair. Even if your shoes still look good, they lose their cushioning effects after approximately 750 miles. After that point, the midsole section that pro-

vides shock absorbency wears out. So don't put off buying a new pair of shoes when you need them; you'll be saving your feet and legs.

• *Dress comfortably, but properly.* Socks that are thin at the bottom will not protect your feet and may even cause blistering. Many well-cushioned choices are available in sports stores. These stores also carry lightweight running clothing for keeping warm and dry in the winter, and cool in the summer. A hat and mittens are essentials on a cold winter's day. In the summer, a thin hat will shade your head from the sun and help prevent heat reactions.

• *Choose running surfaces that minimize shock and stress.* To minimize harsh effects on your body, choose to run on grass and earth whenever possible. If these conditions are unavailable, choose asphalt roads over concrete pavements. Another tip to the road-runner: Take the contour of the road into consideration. What I mean is, sometimes the shoulder of the road is slightly lower than the center, which can result in one leg touching a lower surface than the other. This can cause an imbalanced torso. To prevent this from happening, look for a flatter road, or one that is less traveled. Usually, you want to run facing traffic, but on a road that is not often used, you may be able to run on either side, evening out the effects of the slope.

### 129 Runners: Seek green.

Remember when your mother told you not to play in traffic? Good advice, and you shouldn't run in or with traffic either. I see people do this all the time, but it's really a practice to be avoided. Running alongside heavy traffic can undo all your good intentions in that a half hour's activity in a polluted urban environment can cause you to breathe in as many toxins as you would get from half a pack of cigarettes. (Of course you wouldn't actually be *smoking* the things, would you!? That's personal pollution, big-time.)

If you live in the city, work out in the park whenever possible. The trees will shield you somewhat from the harmful effects of air pollution.

## 130 Never underrate walking.

Walking's first virtue: You can do it anywhere—and you should! Walking provides the same benefits as running, although you do have to do it for a longer period of time. But the big plus is that it's a gentler form of conditioning, one that people of all ages and at all levels of physical conditioning can perform. That's why doctors generally recommend this form of exercise to their patients.

As you'd do with running, take your pulse before you start, step down as you move from heel to toe, and swing your arms naturally. Do not carry anything in your pockets that unbalances you, and never keep your hands in your pockets or pressed to your sides. Walk with a rhythmic gait. Again, grass and earth are the best places for walking, but any surface will do, indoors or out. Some people even set up an aerobic walking course for themselves in shopping malls; it's certainly better for your body than hanging out in shopping mall food courts!

As you schedule walking into your life, remember that you do need to walk for a longer period of time to achieve the same cardiovascular effects as you would from running. So begin walking for 20 to 30 minutes, and during the next few weeks, up your time by 10 minutes weekly until you reach 90 minutes. Gradually build up to your target heart rate and check your pulse every 10 minutes to see if you are working at that level.

**THE HOWS AND WHYS OF EXERCISE**

### 131 More power to ya! Try power walking or racewalking.

For a revved-up walking routine, try power walking (racewalking's the same thing, only faster). If you've seen people walking superfast, as if they were churning through the air, that's power walking, and it's a great aerobic exercise. It looks like the person wants to run, but it's not a run—one foot's always on the ground. The right way to do it: The body's leaning forward from the ankles, at about 5 degrees, to compensate for gravity. Ears are aligned with shoulders; you're not craning your neck. Arms are at right angles, as if you're giving someone an upper cut, and they're pumping vigorously.

And here's the real secret to getting oomph and speed into your racewalk—you rotate a hip slightly forward with each step, in order to extend your stride. You may look a bit like you're doing the rumba, or a Marilyn Monroe impersonation, but the extra inches you get out of each step really add up in terms of distance covered over time. Once you get the hip action down, you'll be moving forward like a dynamo and getting a super workout at the same time.

### 132 Do the exercise that gets you someplace fast—cycling.

Bicycle riding is an excellent complement to running; it gets you to use front leg muscles, while running employs muscles in the back of the legs.

For the best cardiovascular conditioning, ride at an even pace that places your heart in the middle of its target range. If your pace is too slow or too hard, you will achieve less of an effect. To improve speed and stamina, try interval training. Sprint for 30 seconds, then ride at your normal speed for 30 seconds. Do this three to five times in a row. After your workout, stretch your legs.

(Interval training, which we'll discuss more soon, can be used in any aerobic activity. It refers to varying the speed and distance of an activity, either within one workout or from one session to the next. So if you run, for instance, you would alternate a shorter, faster run, or "speed burst," with a longer, slower "recovery" run. Or one day you would jog, and the next, run for speed.)

Good-quality biking shoes will protect your feet and legs from the force of pedaling. The second-best choice is a running or walking shoe. Pant clips can keep your clothes from becoming tangled in the chain. As for the bike itself, use one with a solid frame that is right for your height. Women often ride men's bikes, as their center crossbars make them more stable. And while racing bikes look nifty, leave those low-down handlebars to racers only, because they contort body position too much for the average person.

Adjust the seat to the height that is correct for you, the level at which your knees are only slightly bent when the pedals are at their lowest. If you ride at night, wear light-colored clothes and place a red reflector on the back of your bike.

Indoors, the same general rules apply. Keep handlebars straight for better alignment and less strain on the lower back. And don't slack off just because you're in your living room watching the soaps! You will only achieve good effects when you work at your target heart range.

### 133 Enjoy life in the lap lane.

Welcome to waterworld—your local pool, that is! Swimming's the one exercise that gets you totally out of your element and immerses you in another.

Many people swear by it, because it's relaxing, refreshing, and has so many bodily benefits.

It's aerobic, of course. Plus swimming increases flexibility while building up arms, shoulders, and rear leg muscles. Pressure on bones and joints is minimal, making the activity ideal for people who are injured or who have structural problems.

Can't swim? Your "Y" gives lessons, and it's really rewarding to finally get the knack of this skill. But if that's not your cup of tea (or chlorinated water!) you can still benefit from the pool by going in up to waist level and then walking slowly from one side to the other. Take your pulse before starting to water-walk, and build to your target heart rate for 20 to 60 minutes.

Deep-water running is another aquatic option for building strong legs. (Swimmers only, please.) Wearing a special life vest, you "run" across the deep end of the pool. At first you may be able to keep this up for only 1 or 2 minutes, but your goal should be 30 minutes. Deep-water running can be a supplement to a running program, or a way to heal from an injury that requires building muscle strength.

Swimmers, like runners, need to work out 20 to 30 minutes, 3 to 5 days a week. First, follow the pre-exercise routine described earlier. Then begin with an easy stroke, such as a side stroke, and gradually change to a more challenging one that builds you up to your target heart rate. If your routine becomes too demanding, swim on your back; if you need more of a challenge, try the butterfly stroke.

Interval training can also be used to increase speed and endurance. Sprint for 30 seconds, and swim normally for 30 seconds. Repeat this pattern three to five times. Refrain from swimming one to two days a week to help your leg muscles recover from stress.

If you're swimming in a pool, the best water temperatures for your body are between 77 and 81 degrees F. A bathing cap or ear plugs and goggles can prevent ear infections and conjunctivitis. Avoid pools that use excessive amounts of chlorine, because this chemical can have an adverse effect on your blood chemistry.

*Note for ocean swimmers:* The ocean is a beautiful place to swim, but you must respect its power. An undertow can unexpectedly pull you far out in seconds. If this should happen, don't panic or fight the current. The undertow's force will lessen further out. Then, you can swim diagonally, not straight, back to shore.

### 134 Feel like a kid again—get out the old jump rope!

Jumping rope will bring you mentally back to your playground days, and physically back to a more youthful condition, if you do it right. Rope jumping has some great benefits, especially for dieters. You can burn more calories per minute than you can with any other form of aerobic exercise. This exercise is also great if you travel. Packing a rope is simple, and jumping can be performed in any small space. But there is danger attached to this activity as well. If you start out too strenuously, you can injure your lower back and legs.

The way to begin is slowly. Jumping is tough to do. If you are already in good condition, start out with a 2- to 4-minute routine. If you are heavier or older, do less. Start by running or walking in place. Walk or run in place until your feet come off the ground at a fast pace. Then jump on both feet at the same time for 10 to 30 seconds, with or without rope. Be light-footed; never pound the ground. Rest by walking in place for a few minutes. When you catch your breath, repeat the process. This is a form of interval training.

Do not jump every day; it's too hard on your feet and legs. Every two weeks boost your time by a few minutes. Your ultimate goal is 20 to 30 minutes.

## 135 Look at these other aerobic choices.

Aerobic activities are everywhere, if you're looking. Consider these:

• *The skiing that anyone can do—cross-country*. Imagine yourself in the midst of a winter wonderland of snow, trees, and fresh, crisp air. All you hear is the whoosh of your skis against the powder. Sounds wonderful, but who wants to risk life and limb hurtling down a slippery slope at some breakneck speed?

Here's the great news: You don't have to go fast to ski, if you do it cross-country style. You don't even have to go down hills if you don't want to, because you can reap a lot of the benefits of cross-country skiing just by gliding along level ground. In short, you can tailor your cross-country ski routine for whatever adventure and fitness level you're at, and get a super workout doing it.

This exercise is considered superior to a lot of others because it works both upper-body and lower-body muscles. You can enjoy this sport outdoors during skiing season, or indoors year-round, using a machine.

Note that if you do take to the hills with cross-country, you'll be making your own way uphill on your skis, rather than taking lifts, as with downhill skiing. As you "herringbone" your way up the steeper inclines, you'll be getting a bonus workout.

• *Row, row, row toward health*. Can't afford a yacht or fancy powerboat? Who needs 'em, when you can traverse the water with old-fashioned oar-power and get aerobically fit at the same time! Being out on the water is a soothing experience that can really make your day, and boost your fitness level at the same time. But if you're beached, you can still "row," with a machine. Arms, leg muscles, back, and abdominals will all benefit, in addition to your heart and lungs.

• *Shall we dance? Aerobically, of course.* For those who are energized by music, aerobic dancing is great fun. The camaraderie of a group is motivational for some people, although you certainly don't need others to dance. A videocassette can guide you at home, and if you're inventive you can use it as a takeoff point for developing your own personalized routines.

• *Other aerobic activities.* You might like to try roller skating, rollerblading, step routines, a mini-trampoline (also known as rebound jogging), or a treadmill. Aerobic effects can also come from tennis, handball, racquet ball, squash, and basketball.

In case you're wondering, baseball and softball won't do much for you aerobically. Some people assume that baseball, with its wholesome, all-American image, is a healthful activity to engage in. But baseball's really a sport, rather than an exercise. That's because you're not usually doing much while engaging in the game. So aerobic, it isn't.

## 136 As you advance in fitness, try interval training.

This technique, used by the pros to build speed and endurance, combines aerobic and anaerobic exercise. Basically, while performing an aerobic activity you're sprinkling in some sprints.

Here's what you do: Begin with an aerobic exercise, such as walking, running, cycling, or swimming. After a few minutes at a moderate rate, get your heart rate close to the top of its target range. (To review, you subtract your age from 220; your target range is between 60 and 80 percent of that number.) You work at that top-of-the-range pace for 30 to 60 seconds. Then you ease up until your heart rate drops to about 70 percent of its maximum (this is the middle of your target range). Follow the sequence three to five times. Do not drop below your target range minimum—60 percent—or you will lose this technique's benefits.

After you become used to this method, you can challenge yourself further by increasing the number of sequences, or the intensity or length of the sprint. In addition, the rest period can be shortened.

### 137 Finished with your aerobics? Don't stop now!

Don't be deceived by the loose and limber feeling you get right after working out. Exercise tightens muscle fibers, and you need a post-exercise routine to get them back to their natural length. This will prevent injuries. In addition, you need to cool down so that your pulse returns to normal.

So be cool and heed the first rule of cool-down: *Never just stop.* Sure, you're done with your aerobic activity, but you don't want to shock your system by becoming suddenly immobile. The best thing to do? Walk. Walking around slowly for a few minutes will help ease your body's transition out of it's heated, revved-up state.

You see, what you're trying to do immediately post-exercise is cool the body down and slow the heart rate. You want the blood that has flowed to the extremities to return to the heart. To do this, keep moving until your heart rate is within about

20 beats of its normal resting rate. Continued moderate movement allows the muscles to do the work of getting blood back to the heart.

After you've moved slowly for a short period and your heart rate is moderating, it's time to stretch. You'll probably need between 10 and 30 minutes of stretching. If your muscles are still tight the following day, your body is telling you that you need to stretch some more.

Some rules to remember: As with pre-exercise stretches, post-exercise stretches must be done gently. Perform each exercise 3 to 5 times, and hold for 20 to 30 seconds. Keep breathing as you hold your stretch. Be aware of any strained muscles, and do not stretch into a muscle that is hurting you.

Here are a few basic stretches for the legs and buttocks:

**REAR LEG MUSCLES.** Stand facing a wall, close enough to almost touch it. Your feet should be shoulder-width apart. Hold the palms of your hands against the wall, at about face level or higher. Take a step straight back with one leg. (Make sure that the foot is still at shoulder width, not angled in.) Keep the front knee bent at about a 90-degree angle. Lean forward to stretch the back leg, supporting yourself with your hands and forearms. Keep your back knee straight, and your front knee bent.

Now your elbows are against the wall, with your face between them. You should feel the stretch in your lower rear leg, up to the point just above the knee. Be careful not to hyperextend the knee by throwing your hips too far forward. Your foot should be positioned at the point where your heel will just stay on the ground when you lean forward.

Finish the stretch by pushing out with your hands and moving your foot back slightly to the next farthest point that it will stay on the ground. This stretches the muscles a bit more, allowing you to repeat the exercise with your leg positioned farther back. If your heel rises up when you lean forward, move your foot slightly closer to the wall. Repeat the stretch 5 times for each leg.

**MID-CALF.** This is a variation of the above exercise. Here the back leg should be slightly bent forward at the knee to stretch the soleus muscle in the mid-calf. Once again, repeat the stretch 5 times for each leg.

**HAMSTRINGS AND BUTTOCKS.** Exercising these muscles helps prevent lower-back and knee injuries. When tight, the large muscles in the back of your upper leg exert pressure on your back and shorten your stride. Therefore, these exercises are particularly important.

Lie on your back, lifting one leg into the air, and placing your hands around your calf muscles. Gently pull your knee toward your forehead without lifting your head from the ground. Keep your leg straight, and only stretch as far as it will comfortably go. Depending on the angle, the stretch will affect different parts of the hamstring muscles. Hold for 20 seconds and then slowly lower your leg. Repeat 3 to 5 times on each side.

**QUADRICEPS.** To stretch the muscles in the front of the thighs, lie on your stomach, bending one knee toward your buttock. Then reach behind you with both hands to grasp the ankle. Press your heel down toward your buttock, holding the extension for 20 seconds.

An alternative is to use the standing-quadriceps stretch described in the pre-exercise section. This time, both thighs should be even.

**GROIN.** To stretch the inner thigh and groin area, sit on the floor, bend both knees outward, and put the soles of your feet together. Position both hands on your ankles, and use your elbows to apply a continuous pressure on the knees. Do not bounce your legs; simply try to get the outside of your knees to touch the ground. Hold the extension for 20 seconds and then bring your knees together. Repeat 5 times.

**ILIOTIBIAL BAND.** This is an exercise for people who inflame the ligament that stabilizes the knee. Others can skip this one. To begin, stand with one shoulder against a wall, then step away with both feet. Now cross your feet and allow your hips to curve gently toward the wall, so your body looks like the letter *C* in reverse. Switch shoulders and repeat for the other knee. Do this exercise 3 to 5 times per leg.

## 138 Cool it down, write it up.

During the cool-down period, you should rehydrate yourself by drinking liquids. Do not take a hot shower, or enter a sauna or whirlpool, as this will prevent blood from returning to the heart.

Your cool-down time is an excellent time for logging. No, I'm not suggesting transporting timber downriver—you've done enough aerobics for awhile!—I'm referring to your filling out an exercise log.

Keeping a notebook to record your experiences during exercise is a rewarding activity because you get to see your progress in number form, on paper, in addition to seeing and feeling it in your body. Record how many miles you ran, or laps you swam. Record how long it took you to cool down to your resting heart rate. But don't stop with simple measurements. You can also use this space to write about feelings and thoughts. In so doing, you'll be using your exercise journal to help you grow on several levels.

Here is an example of what a logbook work sheet looks like. Feel free to use this format or to adapt it to measure exactly what you want to measure—the number of minutes you jumped rope, total laps swum, time spent on the cross-country ski course, number of times you rowed across the lake. The choice is yours—as are the benefits.

**LOGBOOK WORK SHEET**

Date_____

Time _____

Resting pulse rate, before exercising _____

Pulse rate after exercising:

at 6 minutes _____

at 8 minutes _____

at 10 minutes _____

Time needed to return to resting pulse rate _____

Energy level (+1, +2, +3, +4, +5) _____

Location_____

Weather _____

Terrain _____

Time elapsed _____

Total miles run_____

Comments (thoughts, feelings, ideas, discomforts, pains,etc.)_____

_____

_____

**139** **Measure your recovery time after exercise.**

As we've mentioned, during exercise, your pulse count should fall within your target range. Once you stop moving, you should be measuring your recovery time, the amount of time it takes for your heart to return to its resting heart rate.

**SUPERCHARGE YOUR HEALTH!**

How do you determine your resting rate? Take your pulse for one minute after you have been sitting quietly for at least 15 minutes. The average resting pulse rate for men is 72; for women, 80. If you are in very good condition, these numbers will be lower, perhaps as low as 60 in men, and 65 to 70 in women.

As you can see from this table, the amount of time it takes for you to return to your resting heart rate determines your level of fitness:

**LEVEL OF FITNESS AS INDICATED BY
RECOVERY TIME**

| | |
|---|---|
| 6 to 8 minutes | good condition |
| 8 to 10 minutes | fair condition |
| over 10 minutes | poor condition |

With regular aerobic exercise, your recovery time will lessen, and your resting heart rate will decrease as well, proof of your improved fitness.

### 140 Cross-train for the most gain.

Perhaps you've started doing an aerobic activity regularly and like the results. Now you'd like to get even better results, and you're ready for more of a challenge, too. Then it's time to mix it up—that is, to cross-train. In cross-training, you do different exercises on different days. For instance, once a week you bike ride. That works on front leg muscles that wouldn't be affected if you were jogging or doing other exercises. Another day you go to the gym and concentrate on building the upper body. Afterwards, you power walk to build strong back leg muscles. With cross-training, you're getting the most you possibly can from exercising.

To put together a cross-training program, choose one aerobic exercise that you enjoy doing and that fits your exercise goals, capabilities, and lifestyle. Pick one that will motivate you to stay with your routine. Supplement your first choice with a second aerobic activity, or with an anaerobic one. This will help you to build and tone different muscles. Running and bicycle riding are two aerobic choices that complement each other nicely. Both provide cardiovascular conditioning yet develop different leg muscles. Weight lifting is a good anaerobic option for strengthening muscles, and thus lessening your chance of injury.

No matter how anxious you are to see results, start slowly with a new activity and gradually build up. Doing too much too soon can harm your body and ultimately slow you down. Perform your activity for 20 minutes per session during the first four weeks. Then increase by 10 percent every two weeks until you reach your maximum time limit for the activity. Ten percent of 20 minutes is just 2 minutes, but that's the successful athlete's way of adding time—in small increments. If you have heart problems or are over 35, increase your time by 10 percent every four weeks instead of two.

Remember to perform anaerobics before aerobics, if you're doing these activities on the same day. Also, you should allow at least 48 hours to elapse between anaerobic workouts, because your body needs this time for tissue repair.

### 141 Work out with weights.

What are you weighting for? Weight training is a good anaerobic complement to an aerobics program. By increasing muscle flexibility and strength, you lessen your risk of injury from weak muscles. You can also build muscles not used in your primary workout. If you run, for instance, you have strong rear leg muscles, and may want to focus on the development of arm, shoulder, and anterior leg muscles through weight training.

If you haven't gotten involved in weight training yet, you probably associate this activity with huge Mr.-America-type muscles. But this should not be your goal. The added weight of such muscles would only prove burdensome to your aerobics routine. Focus instead on exercises that improve strength, flexibility, and range of motion. You don't need tight muscles slowing you down.

Here are some weight training tips.

• *Anaerobics before aerobics.* If you are lifting weights and performing an aerobic activity on the same day, remember to lift weights *before* an aerobics routine, never afterwards.

• *Warm up and cool down.* Before your training session, start with a 10-minute warm-up. Using a stationery bike or treadmill, or running in place, can help you get started. Then stretch your entire body, as we've described in the section on warm-ups. Afterwards, stretch to cool down. These precautions will help you avoid muscle injury. Additionally, stretching after your workout will lessen the amount of soreness you experience during the next few days.

• *Begin with moderate weights.* They should be easy enough to handle, yet tough enough to make you tired toward the end of each set. The first repetitions (reps) within the set tone muscles; the last more difficult ones build strength. Most improvement occurs at the point of muscle fatigue; therefore, once you can perform your final two reps with ease, increase weights by 2.5 to 10 pounds.

• *Set conditioning goals.* The type of benefit you receive depends on the amount of weight and the number of reps. Fewer reps (8–10) with heavier weights build muscle mass while more reps (12–15) with lighter weights improve tone and increase strength.

• *Use good form.* Each rep should be performed slowly, with good form. Squeeze the muscle when it is contracted, and stretch the muscle in its reverse position. Fight the urge to simply run through each set; treat each set as 8 to 15 separate reps.

Note that free weights provide the same benefits as machines, but help to develop better coordination. The one danger is that they can fall. Working with a partner can increase your safety margin.

• *Rest between sessions.* Rest between workouts is essential. Weight training breaks muscles down, and it takes 48 hours for them to repair themselves. So do allow at least 48 hours to lapse between weight training sessions.

### 142 Do these exercises for specific muscles.

The following exercises, most of which use weights, can be used to build up various muscles:

**CHEST: DUMBBELL FLIES.** With elbows slightly bent, hold two dumbbells at arm's length above the chest. As you spread the arms to the sides, stretch the chest muscles. Stop when elbows are at body level, and return to starting point. Do 15 reps.

**SHOULDERS: MILITARY PRESS.** Sitting in a chair, grip a barbell with a shoulder-width grip. Hold at chin level. Lift overhead to the point of complete extension, then return to starting position. This exercise can also be done with dumbbells. Do 15 reps.

**TRICEPS: SEATED DUMBBELL FRENCH PRESS.** Sitting on a bench with back support, hold a dumbbell vertically with palms flat against the weight. Raise arms up and slightly back until they are fully extended. As you bend your elbow, slowly lower dumbbell behind head and neck. You should feel a stretch in the triceps as you do this. Extend weight back up to starting position. Do 12 to 15 reps.

**HAMSTRINGS: STIFF-LEGGED DEADLIFTS.** Stand with feet together. Hold barbell with arms hanging down in front of you. With shoulders back and head up, bend at the waist, and allow weight to hang down in front of you. Your hamstrings will stretch in the process. Return to starting position. Do 12 reps.

**ABDOMINALS: CRUNCHES.** Lying with your back on the floor, place hands on shoulders or across the chest as you lift from shoulders. Do not lift lower back. At your highest point, squeeze abdominals. Work up to 3 sets of 20 reps.

**BACK: FRONT LATERAL PULLDOWNS.** On a high pulley machine, reach above head and grip bar. Pull down to top of chest area and return. Do 15 reps.

**TRAPEZIUS: DUMBBELL KICKBACKS.** Stand with upper body bent forward at a 45-degree angle. Keep one arm against a bench for support. The other arm should be holding a dumbbell parallel to the upper body and facing the body. Raise weight back until triceps is fully extended. Return to starting position. Do 15 reps each side.

**QUADRICEPS: LEG EXTENSIONS.** On leg extension machine extend legs from bent position to straight position, and squeeze muscle. Return to original position. Do 12 to 15 reps.

**CALVES: DONKEY CALF RAISES.** Using donkey calf machine, place balls of feet on platform with heels hanging off edge. Raise up on toes, squeezing heels for maximum stretch. Do 15 reps.

**BICEPS: BARBELL CURLS.** Grip barbell at hip-height and shoulder-width, and bring near chin by bending elbows and keeping them back as much as possible. Lower to starting position. Do 12 reps.

*THE HOWS AND WHYS OF EXERCISE*

### 143 Look at some activities that offer anaerobic plus aerobic benefits.

The racket sports are fun. And you should know that tennis, squash, racketball, handball, and paddleball combine aerobic and anaerobic benefits. The short bursts of energy you need to serve require power and are anaerobic, while the long volleys provide aerobic advantages.

Here's what you need to get started: a court to play on, a good instructor who can teach you about basic skills, equipment, proper clothing, and other players. Look for people with abilities similar to yours to avoid frustration.

Going now to golf, it's not a major fitness-builder, but it could be part of your exercise "menu" if you understand what it does and doesn't do.

Golf builds coordination and concentration. It is basically anaerobic in that it requires short bursts of energy followed by slow activity or rest. But if you walk briskly rather than cart, you can achieve some aerobic benefit as well.

When learning to play, find an instructor who can teach you about proper form, equipment, and clothing. This way, you don't have to unlearn bad habits. In hot weather, drink plenty of water before, during, and after the game to prevent dehydration.

### 144 To banish bumps and bulges, use spot exercises as an aid—but not as your sole remedy.

Spot exercises for fat reduction, as hyped by women's magazines, are overrated. In and of themselves, they're not going to miraculously reshape you. But if your silhouette is less than slinky, don't despair. As you lose body fat through regular aerobic exercise and sensible eating, those troublesome bulges will shrink. *Then*, you can use spot techniques to shape and tone muscles to give you a leaner look. Think of them as a finishing touch to help you optimize your appearance.

With this in mind, let's see what can be done for that most troublesome of trouble spots, the stomach.

**SIT-UPS.** For the upper abdominal area, bent-knee sit-ups are a good toner. We've already talked about sit-ups as part of a warm-up routine; these you can do separately as spot toners and strengtheners. You can do these (and other spot exercises) daily.

What you do is lie on your back with your knees bent and together, and your feet flat on the ground. Your arms are folded across your chest with your hands touching your shoulders.

To do your sit-up, raise yourself up only a couple of inches. As you go up, exhale; inhale as you go down. Make sure the flat of your back stays on the ground, and remember not to go too far up, because this can strain your lower back.

Do two or three sets of sit-ups, with as many reps as you can until you're fatigued, in each. Rest about 15 seconds between sets. (In case you've missed it, a set consists of several consecutive repetitions, or reps, of the exercise. You will often do two or three sets of an exercise, resting about a quarter minute between sets.)

One last note on sit-ups: Remember the old type you did back in school, in which your feet were extended and you'd fling your body all the way up and over? Well, don't. Forget it. It was an exercise error in that it was risky business for your lower back.

**PUSH-UPS.** Another exercise that's great for tightening stomach muscles is the classic push-up. It's the one you've seen in the movies, with new army recruits having to do a zillion because of some minor infraction. But don't worry, at home you can do considerably fewer to get yourself trim.

The starting position: You're on your belly and holding yourself up off the ground with arms straight (hands are placed shoulder-width apart with palms on the ground). Your legs are straight, with only toes on the ground.

Now, exhale as you lower yourself till your elbows form right angles. Inhale as you push yourself back up all the way to the straight-arm position. Do several sets, doing reps in each to the point of fatigue.

Note: If you have to, you can do push-ups with your knees on the ground until you develop the arm and shoulder strength to do classic push-ups.

**LEG RAISES.** To tone the lower abdominal area, these somewhat unusual but simple leg raises are safer than other types.

The starting position: Lie on your back with your hands at your sides. Make a toppled-over "L" out of your back and thighs by bringing your knees up. Your lower legs should now be parallel to the floor.

Now bring your knees a few inches (only a few!) toward your head and then move them forward to form the original "L" again. That's the exercise. Do several sets of as many reps as you can in each.

### 145 Take four steps toward more shapely legs.

Step 1: Lose excess fat.

Step 2: Use very light ankle weights (2 to 3 pounds). Sit on a counter or a solid table. Sit near the edge, with your legs dangling. Straighten your legs, with ankle weights attached, and then lower your feet, doing three sets of as many reps as you can. This will strengthen the quadriceps—the muscles in the front of your legs.

*SUPERCHARGE YOUR HEALTH!*

Step 3: For the hamstrings, lay on your belly. Grab one heel and bring it toward your buttocks, and then let it down again. Do several repetitions, alternating sides.

Step 4: Now on to the calf. These toe raises are simplicity itself. Stand. Raise yourself up onto the balls of your feet. Go back down. Do three sets of as many reps as you can, and you're on your way to shapelier calves.

Note: Don't cramp your style—stretch! That is, after doing leg exercises, you should always do stretches to avoid the risk of cramps. See tip 137 for stretches.

### 146 Want to tone your upper arms? Then don't be a dumbbell about dumbbells!

Women often complain about flabby upper arms. Again, if you lose fat all over, you're going to have some amelioration of the problem. For additional toning, working with light dumbbell weights is the way to go.

The problem is, many women fear that if they work with weights they're going to turn into a muscle-bound Mr. Universe. Well, that's one thing you can scratch off your worry list. As adults, we have most of the muscle we'll ever have. Even *men* can't turn themselves into Mr. Universe. Especially with light weights, all you're going to do is tone and strengthen muscles.

Granted, those individuals bent on bulking themselves up can do so to a limited extent by lifting heavy weights with few reps. But light weights used with many reps will build strength and tone, and stop there.

That said, to tone the muscle in front of your upper arm, do biceps curls. Hold a light dumbbell, palm up. With your arm straight out to the side, move your hand up, to the shoulder, and then back to the starting position. You can also do this starting with your arm extended straight forward.

Timing is important. Take 2 seconds or less for the upward movement. But let the downward movement extend for 4 to 6 seconds. Use a second hand, or try the old "One, Mississippi, two, Mississippi . . ." second-counting technique.

Do three sets of biceps curls, performing as many reps as you can in each.

Now for the triceps, the muscles behind the arm. Hold a dumbbell behind your head. (Your wrist will be behind your ear.) Now raise your arm up until fully extended. Then lower the dumbbell again to the behind-the-head position. The key to this one: Keep your elbow forward to really feel that pull on your back-of-the-arm muscles. Don't get lazy and let your elbow go to the side.

Again, do two or three sets, approaching the fatigue point with each.

## 147 Get hip to this hip-reduction strategy.

Your hips have no muscles. Sorry—you can't tone them by exercising. But wait—don't jump off that bridge yet! If you're losing overall body fat, your hips will be decreasing in size. Also, if you have love handles, you can try side bends, although these are actually more for the abdominal area than for the hip area.

There is, though, a kind of "backwards" strategy to a better-looking hip area. If your buttocks are toned and tightened, your hips are going to look better. The key, then, to hip reduction is to improve your "rear-view image."

The exercise for this is real easy. Holding on to a

tabletop or counter, raise yourself up on the balls of your feet (as in toe raises). Now squeeze your buttocks together. Hold for 10 seconds. Relax. Come down to the ground. Repeat several times.

There's no cause for concern, by the way, if you feel a little muscle shaking or quivering with this exercise. That's okay, because it's isometric. An isometric exercise raises muscle tension, but there is no joint movement, and muscle length shortens only very slightly. Don't be fooled by isometrics' go-nowhere look, though. They do tone and strengthen muscles.

## 148 **Be posture-perfect.**

The various parts of your body can all be trim and toned, but if they're not "put together" the right way, in terms of good posture, your body as a whole won't look its best. Posture says a lot about you—about your fitness, your energy level, and your fashion sense, and even about your attitude and level of self-esteem. Here are some posture pointers from Dr. Howard Robins, a New York podiatrist who specializes in sports medicine and exercise physiology.

You've got to *watch your posture*, Dr. Robins says. Literally. That means checking yourself in the mirror, or if you're outside where no mirrors are available, using what Dr. Robins refers to as the "windows of the world"—the windows of parked automobiles or of stores. It may sound vain, but let's be honest, everybody does it—and you may as well know what to check for as you glance at your reflection.

For the first go-round, look at yourself in a good full-length mirror rather than a car or storefront. Look at yourself sideways, in addition to head-on. Now, be objective—are you standing straight? Or, asks Dr. Robins, are you "schlumped," as so many people are?

If so, correct yourself in front of the mirror. Here's how you should stand:

• Your shoulders should be straight and slightly back.

• Your stomach should be in.

• Your chest should be out. (Following this posture directive is particularly important for women, in that you'll be providing support for breast tissue and improving your silhouette instantly.)

• Your feet and legs should be shoulder-width apart.

• Your head should be aligned above your neck, not craning somewhere ahead of it.

A last posture pointer: As a child, were you told to "Stand like a soldier"? Let's amend that. Soldiers have good posture, it's true, but you don't want to be quite that stiff. So think in terms of standing like a soldier at ease. You'll feel and look better with a somewhat relaxed stance.

### 149 Prevent exercise injury.

It's better to prevent an injury than to treat one after the fact. While soreness and other minor problems are bound to occur when you exercise, safety precautions can prevent more serious and chronic damage. Follow these guidelines to keep your exercise program safe:

• Build up your routine slowly. The old adage about never doing too much too fast too soon works well.

• Warm up before doing any strenuous exercise.

• Pay attention to how you perform the exercise. Poor exercise methods can harm your body.

• Make sure you exercise in the proper environment. This means being aware of obstacles in your path, being dressed properly for the temperature, and exercising in the cleanest air available.

• Stretch and cool down after exercise.

• Make sure you allow enough time to complete your whole program without rushing through it.

• Drink plenty of water before, during, and after exercising. Thirst may not be a reliable guide to how much water you need.

• If you are just beginning a new sport, work with a good instructor who can teach you proper form and technique. Remember that it's always easier to learn correctly in the beginning than to unlearn later on.

• You should feel comfortable when you exercise. Never go beyond discomfort to the point of pain.

• For swimmers—don't swim alone. If no one's swimming with you and there's no lifeguard, you should at least have a "dry-land buddy."

• If you do become injured, don't quit exercising altogether. Instead, modify your routine to something you can do safely. Of course, if it's a serious injury, it must be treated. Then find out if some type of exercise will promote healing.

• Never self-diagnose a serious injury or intense or prolonged pain. See a physician who can diagnose the problem and help it heal with the proper therapy. Ignoring an injury may lead to more serious problems later on.

• Wear clothes that give you room to exercise and the comfort you need.

• Take your pulse in the morning, before getting out of bed, to determine your resting heart rate. If it is 2 to 3 beats faster than your average resting rate, ease up on your aerobic workout that day. If it is 5 to 6 beats faster, it means that your body is under stress and you should avoid working out altogether. On these days, do only your pre- and post-exercise routine.

• Be sure to use good-quality equipment. Note: This does not mean that it has to be expensive or new.

• Change your program around so that it doesn't become too repetitive, working all the same muscles in the same way.

## 150 Rest when you need to, and don't overtrain.

If you have been faithful to your training goals, a brief layoff will not really affect you, and it can even be beneficial if you are recuperating from sickness or injury. If you do not train for a week, your benefits decrease very little. From there, though, things start to go downhill until, at 8 weeks, you have lost most of your benefits and have to start all over again.

At the other end of the spectrum, you have to be careful not to overexercise to the point of becoming sore, extremely fatigued, and unable to sleep. If you find that you are drinking too many fluids and that your heart rate is irregular, you may also be training too hard. Remember, taking it slow is always preferable to overtraining. If you suspect you may be overdoing it, slow down and allow your body to heal.

### SIGNS OF OVERTRAINING

Strains
Sprains
Extreme fatigue and weakness
Cramps
Delayed muscular recovery
Dehydration
Cardiac irregularities
Sleeping problems

You should know that there's a condition called sports anemia, caused by too much strenuous exercise. It's a condition that sometimes affects athletes, such as long-distance runners, swimmers, boxers, and football players. If you think you might be affected, see your doctor, who can detect it with a simple blood test.

## 151 Remember that life is exercise, too (or should be).

Do you know folks who get specifically outfitted for walking or jogging, conscientiously go through their paces, but then go home and take the family van two blocks to buy a loaf of bread? I do, and it seems silly, not to mention expensive and wasteful of resources. Why don't people incorporate exercise into their everyday lives? Here are 10 ways you can:

1. What's your next walkable errand? Walk it.
2. Use an old-style "push" lawn mower.
3. Rake leaves instead of using a leaf blower.
4. Do *moderate* snow shoveling; if you have to strain your back or abdominal muscles, this is not the task for you.
5. If you cultivate flowers or shrubs, use a long-handled flower hoe or spade, rather than a short trowel. That way you can work standing, rather than squatting or bent over, and tone your abdominal muscles in the process. Keep your knees slightly bent to avoid lower-back strain.
6. For parents or other caretakers of babies and toddlers: Pushing a carriage or stroller up hills can be a great aerobic workout, if you're up to it. (Some parents have fun running with the special jogging strollers that have come out. It's fun for baby, too.)

7. Play with your kids in the yard or the park.

8. Don't let rain deter you from walking. Get a poncho or hooded rain jacket (umbrellas can cramp your style).

9. Create your own "StairMaster": As you neaten your house, *don't* be efficient and put everything in a basket to be brought upstairs at once. Go up and down repeatedly.

10. If your area's bike-friendly, use a bicycle for errands.

### 152 Let charts challenge you.

Put a chart on the wall illustrating which muscles are getting toned up with each exercise. Or actually chart your progress by keeping track, for each exercise you do, of the number of sets and reps you perform. This is basically a synthesis of what you've been putting in your exercise log. Those numbers are going to go up over the weeks and months, and actually seeing your progress posted on the wall will make you feel great and motivate you further.

To create a different sort of chart of your accomplishments, try the following. Ask someone to make an outline of your body on a large piece of paper, or make an approximate life-size drawing on your own. Place a picture of your face above the body. Then do what fund-raisers do when they start off with a poster "thermometer" at zero that then gradually rises until the colored-in "mercury" reaches its ultimate goal. You can do the same thing with your body. Color in the body a little bit after each exercise session—just a tiny amount—until one year from now the whole figure is completely filled in. At that time, you will be at—or pretty darn near—your ideal weight, strength, and condition.

## 153 Build a support system.

You don't have to join an expensive gym or health club to exercise. You can do a perfectly nice job of it at home, and without a personal trainer, thank you. But exercising at home doesn't necessarily mean going it alone. For many people, an exercise support system is invaluable. So consider creating a network for your body work. Invite friends to exercise with you, at least part of the time. When I was preparing for a marathon recently, it made it so much easier when friends would come over once a week to work out with me. It motivated me for the whole week. When you exercise together, everyone tends to support each other in their efforts. People inspire you, and keep you focused. They keep you on the straight and narrow.

Or consider a buddy system to keep you from cheating. The other person is there to remind you that you need to do certain exercises that you've been avoiding, or to be more consistent with your routine. Let's say you're depressed, or are going through a difficult time, or maybe you're allowing other life issues to bring you down and create anxiety; in all of these cases you may not want to exercise or eat right. A buddy will remind you to "do the right thing." Plus you'll be helping your friend out in the same way.

After your workout, with a buddy or a whole group, make dinner, or go out to dinner. Post-exercise socializing is always fun, because you really feel you've earned it. Of course you're not going to "pig out," but rather have a healthful, nourishing meal, perhaps followed by another, noneating, activity, such as taking a stroll or going to a movie or play. And even if you only rent a movie, no one can call you a couch potato. You've exercised. You deserve it!

Finally, if you don't have any exercise-minded

friends right now and need to find people to work
out with, try looking in the paper or placing an ad
yourself. You might want to advertise a community
workout. You can put a sign up on a community
bulletin board, or a flyer under your neighbors'
doors, to suggest getting together for power walking or jogging. I'm willing to bet that you'll find a
number of people who will say, "Great idea!"

**154** **Don't fall into the trap of thinking
that you have to act, appear,
or perform a certain way at a certain
age.**

For instance, do you believe that people aged,
say, 20 to 50, can run marathons, but those who are
older can't? It's not true; I know people in their 70s
and 80s who finish the New York City marathon
year after year. The problem with these sorts of
beliefs is that they tend to become self-fulfilling
prophecies. You limit yourself—both physically and
in other ways—because you think age is just about
"do it for you." It may not be though, especially if
you've been following an enlightened eating and
exercise plan. Why not forget old notions about
age, and see where life, your fitness routine, and
the way you actually feel take you? You may be
pleasantly surprised.

# INDEX